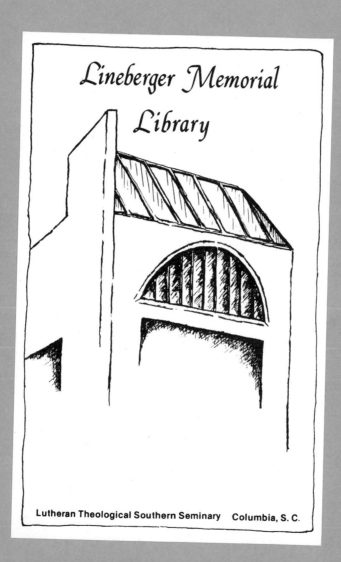

Ethics at the Bedside

ETHICS AT THE BEDSIDE

Edited by

Charles M. Culver, M.D., Ph.D.

Dartmouth College
Published by University Press of New England
Hanover and London

The University Press of New England
is a consortium of universities in New England dedicated to publishing
scholarly and trade works by authors from member campuses and
elsewhere. The New England imprint signifies uniform standards for
publication excellence maintained without exception by the consortium
members. A joint imprint of University Press of New England and a
sponsoring member acknowledges the publishing mission of that university and its support for the dissemination of scholarship throughout the
world. Cited by the American Council of Learned Societies as a model to
be followed, University Press of New England publishes books under its
own imprint and the imprints of

Brandeis University	University of New Hampshire
Brown University	University of Rhode Island
Clark University	Tufts University
University of Connecticut	University of Vermont
Dartmouth College	Wesleyan University

Printed in the United States of America

∞

Library of Congress Cataloging-in-Publication Data

Ethics at the bedside / edited by Charles M. Culver.
    p.   cm.
  ISBN 0–87451–529–7 (alk. paper)
    1. Medical ethics—Case studies. I. Culver, Charles M.
  R724.E82114   1990
  174'.2—dc20
                                 90–38191
                                      CIP

5 4 3 2 1

Contents

Ethics at the Bedside

Introduction

I AM a psychiatrist who has worked in medical ethics for twenty years. For the past eight years I have chaired the Ethics Advisory Committee at Mary Hitchcock Memorial Hospital in Hanover, New Hampshire. Two or three times a month I consult with doctors or nurses at the hospital about cases that raise ethical problems. Some consultations are routine, but others are intellectually fascinating, and a few are dramatic and emotionally draining.

Ethics consultation is a rapidly growing field, but it is a field little known to the general public and not much better known to many doctors and nurses. Ethics consultants see medical practice from a perspective that reveals a great deal about how patients are managed in modern hospitals. The intent of this book is to share that perspective with a general audience.

In June 1988 I sent the following letter to a number of persons whom I knew to be experienced hospital ethics consultants:

Dear ——:

I want to edit a book about the performing of ethics consultations in medicine, and I'm inviting you to be one of the contributors. I want the book to be comprehensible to the intelligent lay reader and also to be of interest to professionals working in the field.

The book will begin with an explanatory stage-setting chapter that I will write. Then ten or twelve experienced ethics consultants will each write a chapter describing in some detail a consultation he or she has performed. I might write a final brief chapter; I would like to decide that after the book takes shape.

The particular case chosen would be largely up to you, though we might need to negotiate a little: it would make no sense, for example, to have three cases involving food and fluid withdrawal in elderly adults. [Editor's note: perhaps because of this admonition, no author dealt with this topic.] A nice mix might be one or two neonatal cases, one pediatric case, and the rest adult. Many cases will, inevitably and appropriately, center around withdrawal of life support, but

1

other topics should be addressed as well: overriding treatment re-
fusals, whether negligent medical practice should be disclosed to
patients who do not know it has occurred, when confidentiality
should be breached, and so forth. You should write about a real case,
with identifying particulars adequately disguised.

A few basic elements should appear in each of the chapters, though
beyond these there can be wide variations in approach. There should
be, first of all, a description of the morally relevant facts of the case,
sufficient in detail to enable readers to form some independent
judgments on their own. The roles and input of any important
persons in the case need to be described, including patient, family,
and involved health care workers.

You should explain what moral concepts and decision-making
processes you used to form the opinion(s) you did. This explanation
need not be terribly lengthy or abstract but should be sufficiently
clear that an intelligent lay reader can follow your reasoning. If any
relevant health law or concern about litigation was a factor that significantly influenced you (or that you conspicuously ignored), that
should be noted as well.

Important interpersonal or psychological aspects of the consultation should also be included; in my experience only rarely does a
consultation involve the unadorned application of moral concepts to
clinical facts. There are almost always interpersonal nuances involved in injecting moral discussion or advice into someone else's
case. Finally, I would like you to say something about what it was like
for you personally to carry out the consultation. Being a consultant
can be quite emotionally engaging. I often become irritated, frightened, satisfied, or sad as a case progresses. Other times I don't get
especially involved. I would like the essays to reflect that personal
dimension.

I want the book to emphasize the work of the individual ethics
consultant, though I realize that some consultants work in various
kinds of tandem with an ethics committee. Consultations are done in
some places by pairs of consultants, though follow-up inquiries are
often directed toward just one of the pair. It would be important to
describe just how you did operate in the case you describe, why you
did so, and how that went.

While you might, as necessary, note occasional citations to the
literature, you should not regard the chapter as a scholarly review of
the area represented by the case. I want you to tell a story, to emphasize the personal experience you had, and extensive use of citations
might tend to detract from the sense of immediacy I hope will come
through.

Chapters should be about 25 to 30 double-spaced typewritten
pages in length. That's very arbitrary; use an amount of space sufficient to say what you want to say. I'll give you suggestions if I think
the material needs to be added to or shortened.

I hope that you'll agree to participate. I am optimistic about this book. There is great interest, lay and professional, in the activity of ethics consultation, but there is no book that makes available for the general reader a sense of the intellectual excitement and occasional drama that the field contains.

Sincerely yours,
Charles M. Culver, M.D., Ph.D.

I sent the letter to fourteen persons. Two declined; the essays of the remaining twelve (along with two coauthors) make up this book.

Ethics and Medicine

Ethical dilemmas in medicine are more conspicuous and more openly discussed than they were ten or twenty years ago. Why is this so? Two factors seem especially important, and both of them are prominent in the essays in this book.

One factor is the increased sophistication of medical technology and medical treatments. Doctors can arrest disease processes that once progressed inexorably, they can temporarily take over the function of one after another failing organ system, and they can permanently replace organs or functions of organs that have been irreversibly lost. These new treatments are two-edged. In some of their applications they are wondrous: persons who once would have died can be kept alive while their underlying illnesses are treated, and they can return to an entirely normal life. But the technology can be overused in a meddlesome and pointless way. An inevitable death can be delayed for weeks or months while the sufferer experiences little more than a foggy and painful existence. A body can be kept alive for months or years although the person who once inhabited that body is gone forever.

A second reason that ethical dilemmas are more conspicuous today is that patients are demanding more of a voice in making decisions about their treatment. Physicians may be less paternalistic than they once were, but old habits die hard. Patients have come to understand that many decisions that doctors make about their care are not "medical" decisions. For example, whether a patient dying of cancer should have another course of toxic chemotherapy very much depends on her values at the time: whether she would prefer to have her painful life end sooner or would prefer to endure the unpleasant side effects of a treatment that might give her some chances of living longer. Different patients in identical medical situations will choose differently. Their values lead them to elect different trade-offs between the quality and the length of their lives. Their doctors cannot know better than they what they themselves prefer.

The field of medical ethics has grown and matured significantly in the past two decades. Useful intellectual analysis has been carried out about many of the troublesome ethical problems that health care workers face. Articles on medical ethics are published frequently in the leading medical journals, and lectures and seminars on medical ethics take place in most medical schools and residency training programs. Most physicians are much better informed about ethical issues than they were ten or fifteen years ago.

Physicians who have had a reasonable exposure to the concepts and decision-making procedures of medical ethics are able to manage adequately the majority of the ethical dilemmas they encounter in their practice. Still, in ethics, as in any discipline, some problems are complex, and it is useful to consult with persons who have studied the subject in depth. For this reason an increasing number of hospitals have available for their staff some form of ethics consultation.

What Is Ethics Consultation?

Ethics consultation in the form this book describes is a new phenomenon. Few persons have been carrying it out for more than ten years, most for much less. Although there are beginning to be ethics committees and ethics consultants available for outpatient settings, most consultation activity is concentrated in hospitals, particularly in large academic referral centers but increasingly in smaller rural and suburban hospitals as well.

Some hospitals have established ethics committees, and as one of their functions, these committees may deliberate about cases that are brought to them. As the number of cases increases, however, it often becomes impractical for the committee as a whole to be quickly or frequently assembled. Therefore, consultations may be carried out by one or two committee members acting alone. In this role they are often referred to as ethics consultants. Consultants may phone other committee members for advice and discussion during a consultation if they feel that would be useful. For example, if a case appears to raise significant legal as well as ethical issues, a lawyer member of the committee might be called. The consultant usually reports the case and its disposition at the next meeting of the ethics committee for discussion and critique.

Who performs consultations? Most consultants are either physicians who have obtained specific training in the concepts and decision-making procedures of medical ethics, or moral philosophers who have obtained training in working in the clinical setting. Of the fourteen ethics consultants writing in this book (two of the twelve papers have two authors), seven have medical degrees and seven do not.

Ethics committees and consultants rarely have any jurisdiction within a hospital; whether they are consulted at all is decided by the doctors and nurses involved with a case. If they are consulted and if they have any advice (they usually do), whether that advice is or is not followed is also up to the involved health care team to decide. Thus, the authority to make decisions remains where it always has been: between the health care team and the patient. In the jargon of the trade, this is referred to as the "optional-optional" model, and it is nearly universally followed. In some instances a department in the hospital may decide always to involve the committee in a certain kind of case—for example, some infant care nurseries always ask for a consultation if they are considering withdrawing life support from a non-terminally ill infant—but that is not a requirement imposed by the ethics committee.

Although a few committees accept consultation requests only from physicians, the majority accept them from any member of the health care team. In some hospitals nurses frequently initiate consultations. Some committees also accept consultations from patients and family members directly and advertise their willingness to do so in informational brochures handed out to patients when they enter the hospital.

The Content of Ethics Consultations

What kinds of issues come to committees and consultants? The great majority—estimates range from 70 to 80 percent—involve the question of withdrawing life support from a gravely ill patient. A large variety of other issues make up the remainder. Here are some examples that have come to the committee I chair: whether to treat a patient who is inexplicably refusing what appears to be a life-necessary treatment; whether to divulge to an elderly, just-widowed woman that she has latent syphilis or instead simply treat her surreptitiously or not at all; whether to inform an unsuspecting wife that her husband has tested positive for the AIDS virus although he does not wish her to know; and whether to inform an unsuspecting family that the brain damage their daughter sustained during surgery was not bad luck but a result of the negligence of the operating team.

But the problem of how and when to allow a patient to die is the most common and perhaps the most arresting of all, and that is the issue about which nearly all of the authors in this book have written.

The Process of Ethics Consultation

What do ethics consultants actually do when they are asked to help with a case? I will return to that question in the Epilogue, after you have read the twelve examples contained in this book, but I want to lay a little groundwork here.

The field of ethics consultation is new enough that there is not yet any general theory of its practice. One important thing that all consultants do is to apply the concepts and decision-making procedures of medical ethics to the facts of a particular case. Most cases require more than that.

Occasional cases are straightforward and limited in scope and can be adequately managed over the telephone with the person making the request, but most cases require in-person investigation by the consultant. It is often necessary to visit the ward, read the patient's chart, talk with the patient if he is competent, and talk with involved family members and members of the health care team. These activities are done to develop a data base of the morally relevant facts. Rarely does the person requesting the consultation have enough of these facts available. This is not a criticism; one must know something about medical ethics to know what facts are and are not morally relevant. Part of the consultant's skill is to develop the data base efficiently; this will be observed time and again in the cases described in this book.

Some consultations can be carried out in one or two hours. Others, like many described here, are more complex and may extend over several days or longer. Sometimes the morally relevant facts of a case change over time; for example, a reasonably optimistic prognosis may change to a very poor one, and what is morally appropriate or inappropriate to do may change in response. Consultants who are called into a case frequently must follow it over time. Ethics consultants, like other hospital consultants, usually document their opinions in the patient's chart. A typical chart note might begin by summarizing the consultant's understanding of the morally relevant facts of the case and then give the consultant's opinion about ethically appropriate ways to proceed.

But, as this book will show, consultants do more than collect facts, form ethical opinions, and write their opinions in charts. They often become active participants as a case develops; sometimes they become major players.

The Results of the Consultation Process

There are few data to answer this obviously important question. Empirical studies of the consultation process are just beginning. There is strong anecdotal and circumstantial evidence that consultation is useful. The majority of larger hospitals and practically all academic medical centers have established ethics committees, which provide case consultation services in one form or another, and consultants typically receive more and more consultation requests as the service becomes known about and used in the hospital.

Some physicians are skeptical about ethics consultation when it is first offered in a hospital. Rare physicians are explicitly hostile: "We've always gotten along without an ethics committee. Why do we suddenly need one? It's just one more bureaucratic interference in the doctor-patient relationship." But the presence of a committee usually proves to be inoffensive: a physician is never required to ask for an ethics consultation and is reasonably free to ignore the committee's presence if he or she wishes. Some physicians welcome ethics consultation from the outset, and some are initially skeptical or hostile, then, having used the service on one occasion, have referred cases ever since.

About the Cases in this Book

The authors in this book are all experienced ethics consultants. They have for the most part chosen complex cases, some of which lasted over a long period. Most authors selected cases they found difficult or anguishing. In some cases the application of relevant ethical theory was critical; in others the focus was as much on interpersonal and psychological issues as on conceptual clarification. One author wrote about the dying of a member of his own family. Two authors asked if they might invite a relative of the patient whose case they described to write about the experience from his or her point of view; these interesting accounts are included. Best of all, the authors did indeed, as my letter of invitation requested, tell a story.

This case involves the family of a dying patient. The consultation process extended over a long period of time and encountered significant difficulties. The authors' discussion of various issues raised by their case is well done and is pertinent to many of the subsequent cases in this book.

"Code Him Until He's Brain Dead!"

John C. Fletcher, Ph.D.

Philip J. Eulie, M.D.

The Case Begins

AT 11:30 P.M. on June 2, 1988, the telephone rang at my home (JCF). I serve as an ethicist at the University of Virginia's (UVA) hospital in Charlottesville. A resident, Dr. Philip Eulie, said, "Are you awake? I'll give you some time if you need it." The light just having been turned out for the night, I said, "Go ahead, I'm listening." Dr. Eulie said, "I have just admitted a gentleman named William Griner to the medical intensive care unit (MICU). He is deeply unconscious. For the last four years he has been lying, minimally responsive, in a nursing home bed. The nursing home staff recognized that he was making very little urine and had a fever. They sent him to the emergency room, where he was found to be in shock and barely breathing. Treatment with antibiotics, intravenous fluids, a breathing tube, and a breathing machine began in the emergency room." He continued, "The

John Fletcher and Philip Eulie are members of the Department of Biomedical Ethics at the University of Virginia Health Sciences Center in Charlottesville, Virginia.

emergency room doctor who admitted the patient stated that the patient's daughter, when asked how aggressive she wanted us to be, answered, 'I want you to code him until he is brain dead!' "

"I then called the daughter, Pam, myself. I talked to her about what was going on, telling her my clinical impression of her father's situation. I told her that he was critically ill, and there was a chance that he could die. I also said that I was concerned that we could not really be helping her father if we tried to revive him if his heart stopped. She then stated that she wanted us to 'code him until he's brain dead!' "

Surprised by this statement, Dr. Eulie told her that it was an unusual request. "Why do you want us to do this?" he asked. She answered, "You don't understand. Our daddy drank a lot when we were children, and he wasn't around much for us. Now that we have him back, we don't want to lose him." Dr. Eulie said that he wanted to understand her views and would like to speak with the family. "It is important that we all meet to discuss your father's care," he said.

At that point Pam said that she, her two sisters, Carole and Debbie, and another relative, would come to the hospital immediately.

After speaking with the daughter, Dr. Eulie called Dr. Katz, a pulmonologist and the MICU attending physician for the month, to discuss the situation. They agreed that an ethics consultation was needed and that Dr. Eulie should call me. In UVA's Department of Medicine, residents take a major responsibility for the care of patients, although the attending is the physician of record and must approve all major decisions.

The resident, the attending, and I had worked together for the previous nine months in the same department. Both physicians were familiar with the goals for an Ethics Consultation Service I was planning. We three had worked together on an earlier case, and Dr. Eulie had visited a new course on medical ethics being offered to medical students and other professional staff of the hospital. Dr. Eulie said to me, "I'd feel better if you were here when they come. I don't think I've ever heard from a family quite like this. There is something pathologic about this situation."

At that time Dr. Eulie's understanding of the patient's situation was as follows: William Griner was a sixty-one-year-old man with a long history of alcohol abuse and estrangement from his family. Four years prior to this admission he had suffered several strokes, which left him unable to communicate and with an arguably marginal ability to understand others. His family at that time assumed the role of his caretaker, and he was admitted to a nearby nursing home. There he continued in this marginal state of existence and during the four years showed no signs of neurological recovery. His daughter Pam said that a speech therapist in the nursing home believed that he might "comprehend some things" and that at times he appeared to pay attention to the therapist when she spoke.

Several months prior to this admission, he was hospitalized on UVA's medical service for an overwhelming infection from his urinary tract. Dr. Eulie was peripherally involved, but another physician on his team was responsible for his care. At that time the issue of how aggressively to treat him was raised with the family, who wished that "everything be done until he has a flat-line EEG." Despite surgery in the interim to correct the anatomic problem that produced the infection, he had developed another bout of urosepsis and was being admitted to this hospital again.

On exam he appeared comatose, with a breathing tube in place. His skin was clammy to the touch and gray and ashen in appearance. His blood pressure was low and his pulse rate very fast. His heart and lungs sounded normal. Examination of his abdomen was remarkable only for tubing that had been inserted through his skin into his bladder to drain his urine because he was not able to urinate on his own. His neurological exam failed to reveal any higher cortical functions. He was unresponsive, and his eyes were unable to track objects or blink to threat. He did, however, have brain stem function, as shown when his pupils constricted to light, and he blinked when the cornea of his eye was touched.

In the MICU, Dr. Eulie added the drug dopamine to help support the patient's blood pressure. Nothing more was done while we waited for the family to arrive.

The Consultation

We met in a drab, cluttered conference room next to the MICU. Besides the four family members there was a chaplain and a nurse assigned to William Griner. After brief introductions we seated ourselves in odd, mismatched chairs. The fluorescent lights gave a dim, green glow that held little promise of illumination for this midnight meeting.

There was tension in the room. I introduced myself, saying, "I'm a minister by background, whose work now is helping with ethical problems that arise in this hospital. Dr. Eulie has asked me to come and help him. He has an ethical problem." I asked Dr. Eulie to describe his ethical problem. He said, "I have a patient who is critically ill and has a negligible chance for any meaningful recovery. But the family wants me to do things that I do not feel are medically appropriate."

I asked the daughters if they also had an ethical problem and if they wanted my help. Pam asked, "Do you have the power to make final decisions about things like this? What is your role?" I answered, "No, I don't have such power. My role is to help everybody involved with your father's care, and you also, to consider the ethical problems and make the most ethically sound decision. I am here to help all of you decide, not to take sides." She looked suspicious, as if a hospital ethicist would always side with whatever physicians wanted. I asked her if the family had an ethical problem. She said, "We do. We want everything done, but the doctors don't believe it will do any good for our daddy." She added that in a previous admission for a stroke in 1985 her father had been on a breathing machine. She said with some vehemence, "The doctors said if they took him off of it, he would die. They did take him off it, but he didn't die. See! They were wrong! And Dr. Eulie could be wrong tonight. We believe that where there is life, there is hope!" I asked each of Pam's sisters if she shared Pam's view. They both said they did. Debbie: "We are together on this." Carole: "We talked about it before coming. I agree with Pam." I asked them if they would like my help. They said that they did want it, but it was hard to see that it would change anything. I asked them if they understood Dr. Eulie's position. Debbie said in an angry voice, "Yes, we understand. He wants to stop everything and let him die. But we won't put up with it. We will go to a lawyer first!"

I turned to Dr. Eulie and asked him if he understood the daughters' position. He said, "I hope that I do. They love their father very much and do not want him to die. They also want us to use all of our medical knowledge and techniques to keep him alive." He spoke gently in a caring voice. It was clear that the daughters heard him. He added, "I must admit, to be honest, that I was hoping that Debbie would tell me on the phone to just keep her daddy comfortable but not to do anything aggressive to prolong his life. But she didn't." I turned to the daughters and asked, "Are any of you angry with Dr. Eulie or with others here?" They said they were not. Debbie said, "I know that Dr. Eulie is trying to understand." I said, "One thing we can agree on, everyone here is interested in what's best for your father. Now let's go to work."

"What Did Your Father Want Done?"

I explained to the group that when patients cannot speak for them-selves, the task is to find out what they *would* want done about life-sustaining treatment, based on any previous statements, written or verbal. "The task is not to do what *we* want but to recall as much as we can about William's preferences and what kind of beliefs he had." The daughters said that William had not only not written any instructions but that they had never talked about "these kind of things together as a family." They talked a little about the problems they had had in early life, about not being a very close family. They recalled their father's drinking problem. "He used to spend weeks in the woods cutting timber. We didn't see him much." Then Debbie said, "When he got sick from strokes, our family came back together." William and his wife had divorced over his drinking problem.

Since no written or verbal instructions were ever left by the patient, the daughters were asked about his religious beliefs to see if these would give any clue about his values. William had not been a member of any denomination. "He was pretty much of a loner," said Pam. When asked about the religious background of the family, Pam said, "We believe in God, but we've never been involved with any church." She also said, "We wouldn't have any trouble if God decided to take him. But we do have trouble with the idea of causing his death by stopping treatments." She said, "I don't even know where I got that idea, about God's way of dying and man's way of dying, but I have it."

I said that if the patient's own wishes were unknown, then the family was the main resource. "The job now is to make decisions with his best interests in mind," I said. "The way we usually think about this notion of 'best interests' is with the idea of benefits and burdens. Together, we will look at each therapy that your father is now receiving and each one that he *could* receive. We will look at these with Dr. Eulie's help and see if we can decide whether they will be helpful or unhelpful to him. If they will be helpful, then there is a duty to provide them. If one or more treatments will be truly burdensome to him, and will not be helpful, then those are *optional*. That means that a real choice exists and that it is acceptable, in our society, not to give optional treatments."

Benefits, Burdens, and Quality of Life

Dr. Eulie explained each treatment that William Griner was then receiving: intravenous fluids, dopamine, broad coverage with antibiotics, and ventilator support for breathing. He said that each treatment might "make medical sense" while the physicians looked for the cause of infection, but he cautioned the family that it might not be possible to find the cause. He also reminded them of the serious neurological deficit that William already had. "We will not be able to do anything about that, and he could very well be much worse. Right now, I can't make any predictions about whether he will even be back to where he was before he got this infection." I pointed out that benefits and burdens each have two sides. Benefits could be a direct contribution to health, for example, an antibiotic that treats an infection and stops it. Even if benefits were not directly available in the health sense, improvements in "quality of life" could be beneficial, especially if added days of life could be meaningful and enjoyed. Burdens are the opposite of benefits. Treatments could cause *more* pain and suffering and actually be harmful to a patient's quality of life. I suggested that there were differences between Dr. Eulie's and the family's ideas of William's quality of life. I reminded them that people differ about how much pain, suffering, and deprivation of mental life they can accept in others. However, in such a situation, physicians and nurses are ethically obliged to defer to the family's wishes unless that causes them such ethical problems that they must decide to withdraw from the case. I asked Dr. Eulie and the nurse if that accurately described their view of what should be done when differences exist about "quality of life." They agreed and said that they would continue to respect the family's wishes.

I asked Dr. Eulie to describe what could be done if William's heart stopped and what he would recommend. He said that chest compressions and electric shocks could be tried to restart the heart. He described how chest compressions were done and said that sometimes ribs were broken in the effort. He recommended that these steps be withheld because at that stage in William Griner's course, they would be futile. Pam said, "We talked about that and we don't want that done. That is 'man's doing something.' We do not want him to linger a long time on machines." I asked Pam if she didn't see a problem with her thinking because "you could make the same statement about the ventilator and anything else that he is now receiving—that is, 'man is doing something.'" She answered, "You are asking us to make decisions to kill him. That is euthanasia or murder. We couldn't live with ourselves if we did that. But if something happens that is unplanned, like his heart stopping, that is God's way of taking him, isn't it?"

Pam's remark about stopping the respirator being "euthanasia or murder" hit some nerves because this step was frequently taken in our medical center, in just this kind of situation, when physicians and family agreed it was justified. I described an act of euthanasia as "killing the patient in the name of mercy with an injection that has the ingredients to do just that—kill quickly." I said that this act was widely regarded as unethical and is illegal in our society. I called attention to ethical statements by national groups that approved either not starting or stopping one or more treatments when the patient is terminally ill and treatment is futile. I suggested that Pam's thinking about a "big difference" between stopping the ventilator (which she called wrong) and not acting to reverse a heart attack (which she called right) were not supported by such statements and needed to be examined.

Despite much time spent in trying to draw a line of moral difference between active euthanasia (by injection) and "allowing to die" (by stopping the respirator), neither Pam nor her sisters was able to *feel* that there was a difference for them. They felt responsible for the choice and remained morally opposed to withdrawing care, on this occasion and until the last day of William's life, nineteen days later.

Stage One and Beyond

Two hours after the meeting began, an agreement emerged that the physicians would (1) continue to do everything now being done, (2) actively seek the cause of William's urosepsis and treat it if possible, (3) write an order saying that "cardioversion and chest compressions are not indicated," and (4) keep in close communication with the family. The family appeared pleased and said that they thought the meeting was "good." Dr. Eulie and the nurse commented later that they felt that as much as possible had been done. Dr. Eulie said, "I have the uncanny feeling that the daughters were trying to harm their father under the guise of doing good." He was responding to a perception he had had from the beginning that the daughters were "acting out" their hidden hostility for a man who had mistreated them as children. I said that, given his view, Dr. Eulie might urge them to get some psychological help if only to examine their feelings about their father, each other, and the loss they were about to suffer. Dr. Eulie did ask a social worker to see the family but not a psychiatrist.

Before leaving the hospital, I wrote the following note in the patient's chart:

> Dr. Eulie asked for consult regarding choices to forego life-sustaining treatment and family's strong desires for aggressive treatment. Met

with four family members, nurse, chaplain, and Dr. Eulie. Family could not recall patient's ever stating what he would want in this situation. They were strongly in favor of continuing all treatment now going. Dr. Eulie explained his recommendation against cardiac resuscitation. They were in agreement about this. Recommendations: (1) review other forms of treatment frequently as to their benefits and burdens, (2) keep in communication with family and make all decisions with them. Dr. Eulie and family are in good communication.

Over the next two weeks, the patient slowly and steadily deteriorated. He was given two antibiotics (cefotaxime and gentamicin) to treat infections presumed to be in his urine and lungs. He had a Swan-Ganz catheter placed in his heart through a vein in his upper chest to take measurements of pressure through the heart into the lung. He continued to have very low blood pressure. Four different types of bacteria were found in cultures of his sputum and blood, and his antibiotics were changed accordingly. His infection and fever persisted throughout his course. He progressed into congestive heart failure and what appeared to be an adult respiratory distress syndrome.

After ten days and another meeting for ethics consultation with family, nurses, and physicians that also included Dr. Katz, the attending, it was decided to stop antibiotics and resume them only if a source of infection was identified. The rationale for stopping antibiotics, as explained by Drs. Eulie and Katz, was that these treatments would have worked by now if they were going to work at all.

The patient continued to have high fevers. Many blood cultures were unrevealing. On the tenth hospital day, his brain stem reflexes were absent. He did not respond to deep pain. The chance that he would ever recover consciousness was very slight. The family still wanted him maintained on the ventilator. His daughters made the same arguments on this occasion as previously, namely, that although "we do not want to see him like this for months and months, we do not feel that we have the right to make this decision. Maybe God will take care of it before then." Dr. Eulie asked a social worker to evaluate and possibly to provide counseling for the family. The social worker wrote the following note:

> As per a family session that lasted two hours and included 3 daughters, primary nurse, attending physician, ethics consultant, intern, and this worker, it is evident that family does not want ventilator removed as long as there is any chance that he can continue to be physically alive. They are willing to accept his death, but they don't

want to feel responsible for it. Part of their belief is based on the idea that if God wants him to die, He will take him whether or not he's on the ventilator, and since in the past their father had a very poor prognosis and survived, they are convinced that they are doing what is right. These beliefs are not necessarily pathological or dysfunctional and in fact have been a useful coping mechanism to them. It may well be detrimental to ask them to give up these beliefs.

This note reveals that the staff's focus of moral concern had shifted entirely from the patient to his daughters. The staff was now afraid of confronting the daughters' ideas and assumptions for fear of "harming" them.

On the nineteenth hospital day, William Griner went into profound heart failure. As the family had wished, no chest compressions or other forms of cardiac resuscitation were done. William Griner died, still on the ventilator.

His family refused to permit an autopsy. When Dr. Eulie and I reported this case in Morning Report, a daily meeting with the chairman and senior house staff officers, I commented that memories of the case left me "feeling unclean." Asked what I meant, I expressed shame at being part of a process in which such hopelessness was prolonged and so many resources expended. I also felt embarrassed at not having called more actively on resources available in the hospital, such as psychiatry and the ethics committee. Dr. Eulie was still concerned about the "pathology" evident to him in the case, involving the family's perhaps unconscious desire to prolong the patient's suffering. Both of us acknowledged significant anger toward the family and agreed that it would have been simple to ask for psychiatric help with these feelings at the time. It is difficult to acknowledge anger, however, when people claim to be acting out of love. The case also took its toll on the morale of nurses and house staff in the MICU.

The total charges in this case were $50,020.25, or $2,632 per day. Medicare reimbursement was the main source of payment.

Discussion

This case was difficult on ethical and interpersonal grounds. Our discussion is mainly about these issues. We also comment briefly on legal and religious aspects of the case.

There was no dispute among the physicians about the medical facts. This dispute was about an ethical problem: ought a ventilator be withdrawn and a hopelessly ill patient be allowed to die? Why was this problem so difficult? Our hypothesis is that there were underlying emotional problems in this family of a dying alcoholic that affected their thinking and interactions with the physicians and the ethics consultant on the case. Because we did not confront these underlying problems more effectively or ask for sufficient help in dealing with them, our work on the ethical problem was probably hampered and was far less than optimal.

Paradigm Case

Ethical concerns and disputes about forgoing life-sustaining treatment are common. Some 80 percent of requests for ethics consultation in the first year of such services at UVA's medical center were about such cases. At the end of the second full year of services, these cases accounted for 66 percent of 123 formal consultations.[1] When an adult patient is mentally capable of refusing such treatment, the case is usually straightforward, even when relatives object. The patient's wishes are respected. When the patient is so ill, impaired, or (as in this case) totally incapacitated and without any advance directives to family or physicians, the case can be far more complex.

"To forgo" has two meanings: either not to start (to withhold) one or more treatments or, having started, to stop (to withdraw) one or more treatments. The withholding option in this case began in the emergency room (ER). This dispute later flowered about withdrawing life supports, but it began as a withholding case. The ER doctor's question, "How aggressive do you want us to be?" framed this option. This way of asking the question is mistaken and sets the stage for subsequent problems. It puts the entire onus of decision making on the family, precludes the doctor from making any recommendation, and is likely to call forth extreme responses (e.g., "Do whatever you think is best, Doctor" or "We want everything done"). Perhaps this case would have unfolded as it did no matter how adroit the ER doctor was. But the initial communication should usually be "Come right away, we need your help in making decisions. Here is what we are doing in the meantime." It is almost always unfair to thrust the issue of "How aggressive should we be?" upon the family, especially before they have had a chance to learn the extent of the medical problems. In the absence of a do-not-resuscitate (DNR) order from the nursing home, which William did not have, the ER physician can make the decision to intubate in an emergency. Treatment such as intubation, which later proves to be futile, can always be subsequently withdrawn.

A case in which *all* family members are opposed to withdrawing treatment, in the face of strong recommendations to do so by physicians, is rare in our experience. More typically one or two family members are opposed to withdrawal among several who are in favor of withdrawal or wavering between the two options. The lone objector may become adamant, threaten to sue, or even bring a lawyer to the hospital. Physicians rarely make decisions to withhold treatment over the objections of family members even when families are irrationally demanding that "everything be done" in irreversible terminal illness where treatment is futile.

But physicians occasionally do act against a family's wishes. Brennan[2] studied decisions to write DNR orders over family objections at the Massachusetts General Hospital (MGH). The MGH has one of the oldest ethics committees in the United States. Brennan found that the Optimum Care Committee, MGH's four-person ethics committee for decisions to forgo life-sustaining treatment, made recommendations to back physicians who wrote DNR orders over family objections in twenty cases in ten years. No families actually sued MGH, although they threatened to sue in at least fifteen of the twenty cases, according to the chairman of the committee, a psychiatrist who has been in this role since its origin.[3] He commented that only by "standing our ground on behalf of the patient" and only by "taking a stand that everybody in the family come in for a meeting in which they are confronted with a decision to write the order" do such families typically come together at all.

Decisions to *withdraw* treatment over the objections of family members are even rarer. We are unaware of any such case in our hospital's recent history. The chairman of the MGH committee could recall only one case in which treatment (ventilator) was withdrawn from a hopelessly ill patient over the objection of a lone family member when other family members strongly favored it. This action followed several weeks of attempts to negotiate. No adverse legal action followed, although the objector's lawyer came to the hospital several times. The lawyer became sympathetic with the physicians' arguments to withdraw.

We regard the case of William Griner as a paradigm, an example that teaches much to remember in future cases, especially in ethical disputes between ICU teams and troubled families about withholding or withdrawing treatment. Among the many problems of troubled families is alcoholism. The surviving family of William Griner, a dying alcoholic, had not yet gained insight into their family history and their own current problems. When preexisting troubles in the family vex the process of medical and ethical decision making, what should be done? In this case, it is likely that the ICU team and the ethics consultant became part of the overall problem, rather than catalysts for insight and motivation to solve problems.

Ethical Problems

We find at least four ethical problems in the case. For reasons of space, we discuss only the first in detail.

Foremost, there was an unresolved dispute about the basis for withdrawing ventilatory support from a patient. Physicians deemed the ventilator to be futile, given the patient's degree of brain damage and an infection that was unresponsive to treatment. The patient's daughters disagreed on grounds they held to have ethical merit. They argued that withdrawal was the moral equivalent of killing. Further, they felt that they, as well as the doctors, would be morally blameworthy for the act. They backed up their position with a religious argument: If their father died from "unplanned" causes, this was acceptable because God would have caused the death; if their father died from "planned" causes, such as withdrawal of treatment, the death would have been humanly caused.

The second problem, really a question, is whether the patient suffered or was harmed by prolongation of futile treatment. Can a patient who has no higher brain function be harmed or suffer?

Third, we find a problem of distributive justice. Expensive medical resources were expended for at least ten days longer than appropriate.

Fourth, is there a duty to confront and intervene in a whole family who irrationally insist that "everything be done" or that nonbeneficial treatment be continued?

Ethical Disputes about Forgoing Life-Sustaining Treatment with Incompetent Patients

Authoritative national groups and the literature in medical ethics have formulated guidance for choices to forgo life-sustaining treatment. The President's Commission for the Study of Ethical Problems in Medicine[4] recommended that "clarity and understanding in this area will be enhanced if laws, judicial opinions, regulations and medical policies speak . . . in terms of the proportionate benefit and burdens of treatment as viewed by particular patients." The benefit/burden standard is ethically derived primarily from the imperatives of the ethical principles of beneficence and proportionality. A Hastings Center Report on ethical guidelines for such cases, representing intensive interdisciplinary work, noted at its outset that "a long tradition of medical ethics acknowledges that the proper goal of medicine is to promote the patient's well-being. In medical ethics this is often called the principle of beneficence."[5] When the patient can no longer be benefited by treatment and may even be harmed, then one ought to rely on the proportionality principle to sort out the relative balances between the benefit and burden of each treatment. This approach was the major ethical framework applied to the case, and the elements of benefit and burden were explained to the family several times. Also, medical ethics literature states clearly that a duty does not exist for physicians to offer treatment they know to be "futile."[6-8] William's physicians and nurses weighed the benefits and burdens, attempting to do so with the help of the family. They recommended not only against using vigorous resuscitative techniques for cardiac arrest but also for cessation of the ventilator, which they knew would lead to death.

If the patient is incapacitated, decision making falls to the proper surrogates, in this case William's daughters, among whom Pam was the spokesperson. The Virginia Natural Death Act,[9] the relevant state law on the subject, requires that next of kin or other legally authorized persons agree about decisions to forgo treatment when an incapacitated patient is terminally ill and has left no advance directives in writing. In the absence of a spouse, the law's requirement is that a "majority of the children reasonably available for consultation" who are present in the decision-making situation must agree to withhold or withdraw treatment.

There is little guidance, beyond formal recommendations, for the resolution of disputes between physicians and families. In a discussion regarding DNR orders for incompetent patients, the President's Commission for the Study of Ethical Problems in Medicine recommended that help for such a dispute be sought by "intra-institutional consultation or ethics committees" but that "during such proceedings, resuscitation should be attempted if cardiac arrest occurs."[10] The Commission recommended the same "fail-safe" process to ensure continued treatment whether the dispute is as it was in this case or its opposite: that is, the family opposes cardiopulmonary resuscitation (CPR) and physicians believe it to be beneficial. In this case, the family eventually agreed to no chest massage or cardioversion. They would not agree to withdrawing the ventilator. We interpret the Commission's guidance in this situation to mean that it would be clearly unethical for physicians to withdraw the ventilator over the family's objections without seeking help for the dispute. To do so would not only violate the surrogate's autonomy but would risk doing unjustified harm to the patient. The Commission advised that "some form of review mechanism within a hospital is generally more appropriate [than a court] for such disagreements," but it recommended going to court for "serious, intractable disagreements between a patient's surrogate and physician."[11]

In our view, the family took an inconsistent ethical position: they were willing to withhold CPR for cardiac arrest but unwilling to withdraw the ventilator. The President's Commission discussed the distinction between withholding and withdrawing in some detail. Conventional wisdom has been that it is harder to withdraw treatment than to withhold it in the first place. In a section on "outworn moral distinctions" the Commission concluded that there was no reason to follow this conventional wisdom. First, treatment once started could be renegotiated along the way and then stopped if it was not helping. Second, they argued that not to stop futile treatment can possibly harm and almost always yields no benefits. William Griner's case was of this type. The Commission gave the following guidance against conventional wisdom:

> Ironically, if there is any call to draw a moral distinction between withholding and withdrawing, it generally cuts the opposite way from the usual formulation: greater justification ought to be required to withhold than to withdraw treatment. Whether a particular treatment will have positive effects is often highly uncertain before the therapy has been tried. If a trial of therapy makes clear that it is not helpful to the patient, this is actual evidence (rather than mere surmise) to support stopping because the therapeutic benefit that earlier was a possibility has been found to be clearly unobtainable.[12]

William's intubation and other treatments could be seen as a "trial of therapy" that failed. This was not strictly true, of course, since it was begun largely at the insistence of his family. The guidance of the President's Commission about the lack of logical and ethical weight in a distinction between withholding and withdrawal was explained to the family many times. They could follow the point, but they could not surmount the idea that to withdraw the ventilator would have been an act *causing* death.

The family's ethical position was based on a claim that there is a substantive difference between acts and omissions that lead to death.

They identified acts of withdrawal and omissions with "man's ways" and "God's ways," respectively, that lead to death. Pam's argument had this premise: an act that leads to death is morally worse than an omission that leads to death. If William had been "allowed to die" by not performing CPR in cardiac arrest, she could accept it. However, to remove the respirator was a wrong option because it would have "wrongfully caused death"; her moral judgment was that to disconnect would mean to kill her father.

The President's Commission also considered the weight of a supposed distinction between actions that lead to death and omissions that lead to death. The Commission took the position that although it believed that most omissions that lead to death in medical practice are acceptable, it did not believe that the moral distinction between that practice and wrongful killing lies in the differences between actions and omissions per se. The Commission found that the distinction was hard to draw in practice. For example, if the respirator had been removed, would the physician have *omitted* to continue the treatment or *acted* to disconnect it? The Commission found that the distinction failed to provide an adequate foundation for the moral and legal evaluation of events leading to death. The basis on which to judge such conduct as good or bad, the Commission argued, rests on other morally significant factors, such as duties owed to patients, the patient's prospects and wishes, and the risks created for someone who acts or who refrains from acting.

According to these criteria, withdrawing treatment would have been acceptable even though it partially contributed to William's death. There was no duty to William to continue futile treatment. His prospects for improvement were nonexistent. The risks for the physicians who would act would be mainly of a legal nature, considering the threats of the family to sue. The cause of his death would have been primarily infection and respiratory failure.

Despite repeated attempts to find ethical common ground with the family to withdraw the ventilator, all attempts to reason about it failed to resolve the dispute.

Was the Patient Harmed? Did He Suffer?

The staff believed that continued treatment harmed the patient and that he suffered. William did not experience any pain or discomfort during most of his last hospitalization because of the degree of his brain damage. The brain damage was caused both by previous strokes and by loss of oxygen in the onset of his terminal illness. One needs to have at least some cortical function in order to experience pain. But William possibly suffered in another meaning of the term.

Suffering also has a larger meaning, discussed by Cassel,[13] as destruction of personhood or "events that threaten the intactness of the person." Suffering can also occur, as Cassel points out, in relation to any aspect of the person, including the "realm of social roles." William suffered mainly in this larger sense; that is, his personhood had been first threatened and then destroyed by alcoholism, strokes, and complications of infections. Most acutely, his intactness as a person was under attack by having to endure a misplaced role. The daughters wanted to keep William in a "patient role." The physicians wanted to place him and his family in the "dying role."[14] The disagreement prolonged his life and, in our view, led to many procedures that were, in fact, needlessly done, even if not experienced by William. Full intensive medical care is demeaning and dehumanizing to a person who is in the dying role. Why keep William in the MICU? If we should be willing to generalize our actions to other similar cases, we would not be willing to do in these cases what was done to William.

Physicians and nurses thought that the patient had no quality of life. His daughters disagreed, projecting some hope for recovery and remembering statements by a speech therapist in the nursing home that William appeared to take note of her presence. McCormick's[15] discussion of quality of life decisions drew the line at "potential for human relationships." He wrote, "There comes a point where an individual's condition itself represents the negation of any truly human—that is, relational—potential." To continue to maintain life when there is no possibility of human relationships is, in McCormick's view, a distortion of values. In William's case, the effect was not so much to cause suffering as to prolong unjustifiably a situation in which everyone was suffering and in which the patient's body and what remained of his personhood was being demeaned and harmed by unnecessary treatment.

Distributive Justice

The costs of medical care are a major problem in the United States. A sizable part of those costs, which are rising, are costs in the last year of life.[16] In this case, the taxpayer bore most of the cost. About 27 percent of Medicare expenditures are allocated to about 50 percent of the beneficiaries, namely, those who died in the previous year. To the extent that cases like these contribute to such costs, more creative and effective measures to intervene can conserve costs. Also, scarce resources were expended for purposes that were not medically indicated. This example, magnified many times, can tell us much about why costs are out of control in the United States and why serious proposals are made to ration medical care, especially intensive care, for the chronically ill elderly.[17]

Duty to Confront and Intervene

Brennan writes, "the touchstone of withdrawal of care from an incompetent patient is the substituted judgment on behalf of the patient, and the presumption must be that the family is best suited to make this decision unless extraordinary circumstances are present."[2] Was this case an exception? Were the daughters the best surrogate decision makers? Were William Griner's best interests being served? In retrospect, we believe that we failed to press this question thoroughly by not activating sufficient institutional resources to help study the question.

What is best for the patient? When harm is being done to a patient by staff acquiescence to irrational wishes of family members to continue treatment, there is a duty, based on the beneficence principle, to confront the family and ask for intervention, if necessary, to interrupt the harmful process. A foundation of medical ethics is, above all, to help, and when help is no longer possible, to avoid doing harm. We believe the example set at the MGH is a good one in its response to just this duty. However, the MGH series concerns confronting troubled families who insisted that futile treatment (CPR) be *started*. Our case involved futile treatment being *continued* at family request.

Interpersonal and Emotional Problems

To confront and intervene is emotionally difficult because it would be done on a premise that family members are not placing the patient's best interests first, even when they claim to be acting out of love. Our memory and experience of working with the patients' daughters is primarily of their defensive behavior and argumentativeness. Although the dynamics of troubled families are not limited to those of alcoholics, we did not thoroughly study the link in this case[18] nor attempt to develop it with the daughters. We kept our anger and responses to it to ourselves, which was clearly a mistake.

We learned these things from Pam and her sisters about their father and their family: William was a "loner" who abused alcohol throughout their lives until his strokes; he was gone for long periods; he was divorced from their mother; they never confronted him or sought professional help about his drinking; no discussion about death or serious illness had ever occurred. After his strokes the daughters would gather in the nursing home to visit him. He could not respond or recognize them. What really occurred during this period? The experience of loss in their childhood was partially compensated for by simple physical presence. But what did they do with their anger and rage over the loss of their childhood and the abuse they suffered? Did their wishes for their father to be punished and die become converted to a "reaction formation," a defense mechanism in which "affects are transformed into their opposites and ambivalence is resolved in the opposite manner from which it arises?"[19] Was their desperate desire to keep him alive at all costs the polar opposite of their unacceptable feelings of wanting him dead? Debbie said, "When he got sick from strokes, our family came back together." Possibly the daughters became close in their care of William, but what could they have received from him during four years in a nursing home?

An objective assessment of the family's psychology was not made by a mental health professional, so our view is speculative. We note with interest that Brennan's first case report[20] about writing DNR orders over family objections also involved the family of an alcoholic patient who eventually died of renal-hepatic syndrome.

There were many opportunities to obtain psychiatric consultation in the case; for example, as soon as Dr. Eulie remarked on the "pathology" in the family. Each meeting with the family presented other chances, especially given their family history. Dr. Eulie urged the family to seek counseling and involved a social worker to see them. The social worker's note essentially reflected her (and the staff's) desire not to confront or intervene. Alternatively, we could have involved a psychiatrist to *help us* with the emotional problems we had in relation to the family: frustration, anger, and resentment at having to do things that appeared to be harmful to the patient. Also, an effort should have been made to move the daughters to seek psychiatric help for themselves. Dr. Eulie could have put his recommendation to the daughters on either a general or specific level: (1) "We can offer you some professional help with your hurt feelings, whether your dad lives or dies. This experience has clearly been very hard for you. We have very good people to help you sort things out emotionally, which is hard for me because I am so involved"; or (2) "Many other adult children of alcoholics have found help simply by talking about their experience. You can start to get help here quite apart from the decisions we must make about William."

Legal and Religious Aspects

We are unaware of any case in which a hospital has sought legal relief from prolonging a patient's life because of irrational desires of a family or its members. In a case that is somewhat parallel, a Missouri Court[21] ordered a ventilator stopped, over the petition of parents to continue it, in a case involving a minor who was deemed to be "brain dead" for more than six months by as many as seven physicians. The parents insisted that "he knows that we are there" and that his "blood pressure elevates . . . when we walk into the room." The parents also believed that "spiritually he has been healed, that it is a matter of time before he awakes and it is God's providence when he will do this." The court found that the patient, Philip Rader, was dead according to the definition of death passed by the Missouri legislature.

The chairman of the MGH committee could recall no cases in which the hospital sought legal relief. He commented that his institution would "never institute legal action against a family," preferring to avoid inviting the poor publicity of a powerful hospital "ganging up" against a family. Intuitively, this is an understandable position, but the effort might be worthwhile in the right case, assuming that the hospital had used all of its resources to resolve the problem.

Another internal resource that we failed to use was the hospital ethics committee. The chairman of the ethics committee is authorized to convene an ad hoc group to consider cases that the Ethics Consultation Service refers to it. We offered the services of the committee to the family at one point if they thought that they were being unfairly pressured to agree to withdraw treatment. What we did not do was to consider the ethics committee as a resource for resolving the case sooner. A desire to compromise with the family was the dominant theme throughout the case. We avoided calling on the ethics committee largely to avoid antagonizing the family and endangering the compromises already achieved. But another strong reason to involve the ethics committee was that I, although acting impartially at the outset of the case, became strongly persuaded in a later stage that withdrawal was the ethically preferable course. Another level of institutional involvement would have restored more impartiality to the later stages of the case.

Pam's threats of a lawsuit are instructive in terms of the experience of the MGH. Standing firm on behalf of the patient dissolved these threats, although one must always reassure families that make such threats that seeking legal relief is their right.

We also did not confront or challenge the religious arguments used by this family. The arguments struck us as their efforts to absolve themselves of responsibility for making decisions in the midst of a real problem of human suffering and its relief. Divine help was invoked, it appeared, to assist in a rationalization of inaction, rather than as a source of courage and strength to face a hard choice. Desperation may have prompted these responses; Pam was honest about not being active in a religious community. However, no argument ought to be above rational criticism. We could have fairly pointed out our inner responses to such arguments that encourage resignation in the face of suffering and evil. This passive spirit is incompatible with Judeo-Christian religious movements that inspire a realistic confrontation with the causes of pain and suffering and avoid an absolutistic approach to ethical problems, especially in the context of kinship and intimate bonds.

Summary

In a case of a dying alcoholic man, his family resisted all attempts to limit treatment or to place him in the "dying role." Ethics consultation was partially successful in reaching compromise on withdrawing some aspects of unnecessary care. However, the family would not accede to withdrawal of a ventilator, and the patient lived at least two weeks longer than was appropriate considering his medical condition. In retrospect, valuable lessons were learned about (1) emotional problems among adult children of alcoholics in the dying situation, (2) the consequences of not using all available institutional resources such as psychiatric consultation and intervention by the hospital ethics committee. The possibility of asking a court to provide relief to the hospital is a remote but possibly realistic alternative in future cases of this type.

Notes

1. J. C. Fletcher and M. Boverman, "Ethics Consultation at the Medical Center of the University of Virginia," *Newsletter of the Society for Bioethics Consultation* 1(1988): 4–6; J. C. Fletcher, "Decisions to forego life-sustaining treatment," *Journal of the Virginia Medical Society* (in press).

2. T. A. Brennan, "Incompetent patients with limited care in the absence of family consent," *Annals of Internal Medicine* 109(1988):819–25.

3. N. Cassem, personal communication, December 30, 1988.

4. President's Commission for the Study of Ethical Problems in Medicine and Biomedical and Behavioral Research, *Decisions to Forego Life-sustaining Treatment* (Washington, D.C.: U.S. Government Printing Office, 1983), 89.

5. Hastings Center, *Guidelines on the Termination of Life-sustaining Treatment and the Care of the Dying* (Bloomington, Ind.: Indiana University Press, 1987), 7.

6. B. Lo and A. R. Jonsen, "Clinical Decisions to Limit Treatment," *Annals of Internal Medicine* 93(1980):764–8.

7. President's Commission for the Study of Ethical Problems in Medicine and Biomedical and Behavioral Research, *Making health care decisions*, Vol 1 (Washington, D.C.: U.S. Government Printing Office, 1982), 43–44.

8. T. Tomlinson and H. Brody, "Ethics and Communication in Do-Not-Resuscitate Orders," *New England Journal of Medicine* 318(1988):43–46.

9. Virginia Natural Death Act, 1983; Virginia Code 54–325, 8:1, 8:2, 8:6.

10. President's Commission, *Decisions to Forego Life-sustaining Treatment*, 246.

11. Ibid, 248.

12. Ibid, 76.

13. E. J. Cassel, "The Nature of Suffering and the Goals of Medicine," *New England Journal of Medicine* 306(1982):639–45.

14. H. Osmond and M. Siegler, "The Dying Role—Its Clinical Importance," *Alabama Journal of Medical Science* 13(1976):313–17.

15. R. A. McCormick, *How Brave a New World?* (Washington, D.C.: Georgetown University Press, 1981), 349.

16. J. C. Fletcher, "Ethics and the Costs of Dying—Revisited," in *Life and Death Issues: Sixth Annual Norfleet Forum*, ed. J. E. Hamner III and B. J. S. Jacobs, Memphis, Tenn.: University of Tennessee, 1986), 129–45.

17. D. Callahan, *Setting Limits: Medical Goals in an Aging Society* (New York: Simon and Schuster, 1987).

18. S. Brown, *Treating Adult Children of Alcoholics: A Developmental Perspective* (New York: John Wiley and Sons, 1988), 102. We did not consider the comment of Brown and other experts (P. Steinglass, L. A. Bennett, S. J. Wolin, and D. Reiss, *The Alcoholic Family* [New York: Basic Books, 1987]) on treatment of families of alcoholics on the "dominance of defensive maneuvers." The characteristics of this defensive adaptation are, according to Brown, denial, control, all-or-none thinking, and the assumption of personal responsibility for the alcoholic's behavior.

19. S. S. Marmer, "Theories of the Mind and Psychopathology," *The Textbook of Psychiatry*, ed. J. A. Talbot, R. E. Hales, and S. C. Yudofsky (Washington, D.C.: American Psychiatric Press, 1988), 136.

20. T. A. Brennan, "Do-Not-Resuscitate Orders for the Incompetent Patient in the Absence of Family Consent," *Law, Medicine, and Health Care* 14(1986):13–19.

21. Nancy White et al. v. St. Joseph Health Center et al.; Circuit Court of Jackson County, Mo., Case No. CV 88–14759, July 7, 1988.

*This case describes a straightforward and effective
consultation that involved explaining an important
conceptual distinction to the family of a dying patient.*

A Philosophical Consultation

Bernard Gert, Ph.D.

IT was about 10 A.M. when I got a call from the resident. I was still at
home because I didn't need to lecture to the introductory philosophy class until 1 P.M., and I had no scheduled appointments before
then. I am a philosopher, not a physician, and my schedule allows for
much more flexibility in the times I have to be in my office. However, I
am on the ethics committee of Mary Hitchcock Hospital, and they
know that I can be reached at home if I am not at my office. I knew that
Dr. Chuck Culver was out of town, so I was not surprised to get the call
requesting my assistance. Chuck is the chairman of the ethics committee and does most of the consulting on individual cases, but when he
goes out of town, I serve as his backup. Also, he sometimes asks me to
accompany him when he thinks a case has some features or complications that I might find interesting.

I have been involved in medical ethics for about fifteen years and
have been doing consultations for almost ten years, but I still have
some difficulty with medical terminology. Thus, I usually try to have
the physician explain matters to me in lay terms. My experience has
been that knowledge of the technical details, though obviously crucial
in making medical decisions, does not seem required in those cases
where physicians request assistance from the ethics committee. In fact,
I find that having physicians describe the case to me in terms that any

Bernard Gert is Professor of Philosophy, Dartmouth College, Hanover, New Hampshire, and Adjunct Professor of Psychiatry, Dartmouth Medical School.

lay person can understand usually helps to clarify the morally relevant facts of the case.

In any event, my description of this case will not include any technical medical terminology but will be given in the kind of lay terms that I used when talking with the resident and with the children of the patient. That will make it unnecessary for me to change many of the features of the case to protect confidentiality, for I shall describe the case in such general terms that the description applies to a great many similar cases. I may change ages and genders, but these changes will make no difference at all to the morally relevant facts.

The resident first described the case to me in the following way. An elderly man, in his late seventies, was permanently unconscious and terminally ill. His children, a son and a daughter, were at the hospital and were insisting that their father be given morphine to alleviate whatever distress he was feeling. The attending physician did not believe that the patient needed any relief from pain and was unwilling to give him morphine. She believed the only effect of giving morphine would be to hasten the patient's death.

I assumed the resident was troubled about what he should do. I asked him what he thought about the propriety of giving the patient morphine. He said that he agreed with the attending physician—as did all the rest of the medical team, including all of the nurses—that morphine was not needed in this case. I told him that I was puzzled about what ethical problem he thought he was facing. He then told me that a consulting psychiatrist thought it would be appropriate to administer morphine and that the family physician also thought it would be appropriate. It turned out, however, that neither of these physicians had seen the patient recently, so it was not clear that there was any current disagreement on the need for morphine to relieve pain.

I was unsure about what he wanted me to do, for it was evident that he was already certain that morphine was not medically indicated. I could not understand why he was calling me at all, and I told him so. Then it became clear that he wanted me to talk to the son and daughter. He had tried talking to them and could not persuade them of the correctness of the medical decision not to administer morphine. He thought they were simply being unreasonable, especially because the hospital staff had agreed to withhold and withdraw all life support, including the IVs that were providing food and fluids. He did not know how to talk to them nor what to say, but he and the nurses were obviously troubled by the continuing pressure by the children to give morphine to their father.

I told him that I would meet with the patient's children at the hospital in one hour, and he was obviously grateful and relieved. At the appointed time I was at the nurse's desk on the floor. A nurse at the desk told me that she had been taking care of the patient and that she, as well as all of the other nurses, agreed that there was no point in giving the patient morphine. They had stopped giving the morphine two days ago, and, like the stopping of food and fluids several days before, the absence of morphine had resulted in absolutely no change in the patient's behavior or lack of it. Breathing had remained the same, and so had all involuntary movements and facial expressions.

I was taken into the patient's room, where his children were waiting for me. They were both in their late fifties and casually, though appropriately, dressed. They had been coming to the hospital every day for more than two weeks and were showing some signs of strain. Their father was lying in the bed, breathing heavily—not quite snoring, but making a noise loud enough to be noticeable. Because the room was fairly small and we would have had to see and hear their father during our conversation, I decided that we should meet in another room. We went in search of an empty room and soon found one just a short way down the hall.

I introduced myself and told them that I was on the ethics committee of the hospital but was not a physician; rather I was a philosopher who worked in medical ethics. They then introduced themselves; both were schoolteachers, one in high school, the other in elementary school. This made me feel quite comfortable because I thought we would be able to talk about the situation without any communication problems. They were indeed quite articulate; they described the situation of their father as follows.

His wife, their mother, had died several years ago. Their father had never quite recovered from her death and had been fairly lonely and unhappy. Two years ago their father had had a serious stroke and had almost died. In fact, he had been quite upset that he had been resuscitated, preferring to die rather than to continue his lonely and unhappy life. He continued to complain about this, particularly with the added burden of the aftereffects of the stroke, and he had told them that if he had another stroke or a heart attack he did not want to be treated. As it happened, he developed cancer, which had progressed to the point where he was now not only terminal but was completely and permanently unconscious. They realized that it was unlikely that their father was feeling any pain or discomfort, but they thought it was possible that he was. They pointed out that his breathing sounded labored and that sometimes he had facial expressions that seemed to indicate discomfort. Because he was going to die anyway, they did not see the point of taking him off morphine. They did not take it as a point against giving morphine that it might hasten their father's death; on the contrary, they regarded the hastening of his death as a positive good.

As I listened to their story, it became quite clear to them that I was in no hurry, that I was prepared to listen to them and to talk to them for as long as was necessary to resolve the problem. This had a very beneficial effect. One of their main complaints was that no one had been willing to sit down and talk over the situation with them. That I was prepared to do so immediately changed my relationship with them from one of adversary to one of friend. They were having a hard time dealing with their father's dying. It was a burden to them to come to the hospital every day for hours on end to sit with their unconscious father, and yet they were sufficiently close to him that it was unthinkable for them not to come. They knew and believed that he would never regain consciousness before he died, and they viewed it as absurd that the doctors and nurses refused to give morphine because it might hasten his death.

We started by talking about the likelihood of their father actually suffering any pain or discomfort. The son was prepared to believe that their father was not suffering at all, but the daughter thought there was some slight possibility that he was suffering. However, when I pointed out to her that there was absolutely no change in his behavior before and after the morphine had been stopped, she admitted that that was correct. Eventually, it became quite clear to all of us that the primary reason for their wanting morphine was to hasten death, that pain relief provided a rationalization for their insisting on the administration of morphine, but neither of them had any firm conviction that their father was actually suffering.

I pointed out to them that the doctors had already agreed to stop food and fluids and that no food or fluids had been given since Friday, and as it was now Tuesday, that meant it was very unlikely that their father would live more than three or four more days. They were somewhat surprised by this. They knew that food and fluids had been stopped, but they claimed that no one had told them how long it would be before their father died. Actually, they had been told that their father would die some time ago, and the doctors had agreed to stop food and fluids only when it seemed clear that he was not going to die as soon as they had predicted. I pointed out to them that they were fortunate to be in our hospital, for in many hospitals the staff might not agree to stop food and fluids without an explicit advance directive from the patient, such as a Living Will, and in some hospitals they might not do so even with an explicit advance directive.

Indeed, I was somewhat surprised that our hospital had agreed to the procedure because the patient had not made out any advance directives explicitly stating that he wanted food and fluids withdrawn in these circumstances. Of course, it would have been difficult for him to do so because New Hampshire's Living Will makes no provision for stopping food and fluids, and the New Hampshire legislature has yet to pass a Durable Power of Attorney for Health Care statute. It turned out that the attending physician had agreed to withhold food and fluids because the family was well known to her, and the family doctor and the consulting psychiatrist, both members of the hospital staff, had confirmed that the patient had continually stated that he wanted to die and did not want anything done that would prolong his life. (He could have nonetheless drawn up a Durable Power of Attorney for Health Care document and left instructions about the withdrawal of food and fluids and other forms of life support, but few persons are yet well informed about this option.)

We then had a discussion about advance directives (i.e., Living Wills and durable powers of attorney), and I advised them to be sure to make out an advance directive stating their wishes and specifically mentioning the stopping of food and fluids. I pointed out to them how lucky they and their father had been that his wishes were known by doctors on the staff and that the hospital had been willing to honor his wishes. They and their children might not be so lucky; that is why I urged them to make out a durable power of attorney and give copies of it to their children, their doctor, their clergyman, and anyone else who they thought might be involved. I also advised them to talk to their physician to see whether or not he was willing to abide by their requests. I pointed out that even if such a document was not legally binding in New Hampshire, the fact that they had discussed the matter with their children and doctor and had obtained their agreement would make it very likely that their requests would be honored.

We then returned to the matter of why the doctors and nurses refused to give their father morphine, especially when they already had
agreed to stop giving him food and fluids. Here I was on familiar
territory. I had written an article with Chuck Culver, "Distinguishing
between Active and Passive Euthanasia," and in the last chapter of my
new book, *Morality: A New Justification of the Moral Rules* (New York:
Oxford University Press, 1988), I had shown how this distinction could
be derived from the moral theory I had presented in the previous
chapters. In both the article and the book I demonstrated a way of
making the distinction between active and passive euthanasia that
resulted in voluntary passive euthanasia being so clearly justified that
it became morally uncontroversial, whereas active euthanasia remained
morally controversial.

According to my theory, morality requires everyone to obey what I
call the moral rules (rules prohibiting killing, causing pain, depriving
of freedom, deceiving, breaking promises, etc.) except when, considering the situation as impartial, rational persons, they would be willing
to allow everyone to break a moral rule in the same circumstances. I
regard this as simply making explicit the rules and procedures we all
use when making moral decisions or moral judgments; thus, I intentionally use the theory when talking about moral issues to those who
are not philosophers. I find that making everything explicit clarifies
thinking, and if there is no disagreement about the facts, this usually
results in agreement among all the parties. Indeed, in all of the years
that I have been on the ethics committee and doing consultations we
have always reached a consensus view. This does not mean that in
every case we all advised the same course of action, for in my account of
morality, impartial, rational persons can sometime disagree on what
they advise. However, when the theory says that only one decision is
morally acceptable, we all agreed on that decision. When the theory
allowed for moral disagreement, we sometimes disagreed; but as we
were an advisory committee, this created no problem. We simply advised the physician that either of two or more alternatives was morally acceptable and that the physician could follow his or her own
intuitions.

In this case the facts were no longer in dispute. The father, terminally
ill and permanently unconscious, was no longer receiving food or
fluids. The question to be answered was whether or not it was morally
acceptable for the doctors or nurses to give the father morphine to
hasten his death. The doctors and nurses had already decided that it

was not morally acceptable. They were prepared to give morphine if they believed that it would alleviate pain or suffering, even if doing so would hasten the death of the patient; however, they were not prepared to give morphine when they believed that its only effect would be to hasten the death of the patient.

The son and daughter said that they did not see why there was any difference between stopping food and fluids and giving morphine since both would result in their father's death. Why wait, when not only did everyone agree that there was no point in keeping their father alive, they had actually taken steps that guaranteed his death. I agreed that if their father was suffering in any way, it might be morally acceptable to give him morphine, even knowing that it would result in his dying sooner. However, we were not dealing with such a case; their father was in no pain. Giving morphine might ease their own suffering but not their father's. Thus, one strong argument for giving morphine was absent: it would not relieve any pain of the patient.

We then talked about the difference between active and passive euthanasia. I pointed out that the clearest cases were those of voluntary euthanasia, where the patient is not only conscious but competent, and he rationally decides that he wants to die. In such situations patients may either *refuse* all life-prolonging measures, including food and fluids, or *request* that the physician administer some drug, such as morphine, to hasten death. I told them that I classified the doctor's abiding by the rational refusal of a competent patient as passive euthanasia and regarded it as not merely morally acceptable but morally required to honor the patient's refusal. Patients who had become incompetent but who had made out advance directives refusing life-prolonging treatment seemed to me to be in the same category. Even though their father had not made out such a directive, his views on the matter were clear and unambiguous and had been confirmed by independent sources; therefore I regarded him as in the same category as someone who had made out an explicit advance directive. Thus, I had no problem at all with the decision to stop food and fluids.

We then had a slight digression on the stopping of food and fluids. They did not have any problem in classifying it as passive euthanasia, but they were concerned about the suffering it would cause. I pointed out that in the case of their father, this problem did not arise because in his unconscious state he did not feel anything. But since we were also talking about their own advance directives, I pointed out that contrary to normal expectations (and to mine when I first heard it), stopping food and fluids is not painful, even if one is fully conscious. One thinks of hunger and especially of thirst as being very painful, but that is not necessarily the case. We know from people who have been on hunger strikes that after the first day they do not feel any unpleasant hunger pangs; in fact, some regard it as rather pleasant. What is normally unpleasant about going without food is that you will die, but in the case of some terminally ill patients, that they will die sooner because of lack of food is not unpleasant, for they want to die.

I pointed out that simply not eating does not usually result in one's dying very quickly; usually one can live for one or two months with nothing but liquids. However, if one stops taking fluids as well, death comes much more quickly, usually within a week. We think of dying of thirst as very unpleasant because we think of someone lost in a desert, lips cracked and blistering. But this picture is inaccurate; it is not the lack of fluids that causes the suffering but being out in the desert. Going without fluids in the hospital may result in some skin dryness, but this is easily taken care of by good nursing care, such as applying ice chips to the lips.

They were very interested in this information, and we talked about how important it was for such information to be more widely known. I admitted that the practical importance of the way I made the distinction between active and passive euthanasia depended on the fact that stopping food and fluids was not painful. If it were painful, I did not think that, despite the philosophical power of my distinction between active and passive euthanasia, it would be of any value in deciding what to do in real cases. If the only available method of passive euthanasia were stopping food and fluids (which is often the case) and if this were painful, then active euthanasia would be a much more compelling option. However, it is not painful, and I expressed my belief that if this were widely known and appreciated, and if it were also known that stopping fluids usually results in death in about a week, then this would lessen the growing pressure for active euthanasia.

They then asked me what was wrong with active euthanasia in a case like their father's. However, active euthanasia is responding to a patient's request, not a patient's refusal. Doctors are not necessarily breaking any moral rule when they refuse to go along with a patient's request. Doctors have no duty to do whatever their patients want them to do, even when the patients are competent and their requests rational. When a patient requests that a doctor kill him, the doctor is not violating any moral rule if he refuses, nor is he violating his duty as a doctor. On the contrary, in this country not only has the American Medical Association said that active euthanasia is not acceptable, but it is also against the law. One can be charged with murder if one kills a person, even with that person's consent. Many doctors and nurses have a strong moral repugnance to killing, and no one would want to require them to go along with a patient request to be killed.

I tried to show them that many people would be very upset if it were known that the hospital had a policy that allowed them to kill people on request. If they were claiming that it was morally acceptable for the hospital staff to kill their father, then they had to be prepared to advocate that everyone know that it was hospital policy. Morality is a public system; that is, it must be known by and acceptable to all those who are governed by it. They could not think it right for the hospital staff to kill their father but wrong to act in the same way with regard to others in similar circumstances, where similar circumstances are determined solely by the morally relevant facts. Given the irreversibility and finality of death and the fact that people are not infallible, would they really favor such a policy? The daughter admitted that if a patient came out and asked her to give him a lethal injection, she would not do so, and she did not want to require anyone else to do so. She was less sure of what she would do if she were at home with her father.

I talked about the importance of looking not only at their particular case but of looking at the policy that would result if what they wanted done were regularly done. They seemed to agree that they would not want such a policy. I talked about the problems a nurse would have if their father happened to die right after he or she began administering the morphine, when the nurse knew that the morphine was not being used for pain relief. That also seemed to affect them, but I thought the most telling argument was the realization that they could not simply look at the consequences of the one particular act of violating the rules against killing and against breaking the law but must consider what would happen if everyone knew that everyone was allowed to break the rules in these same circumstances. Since this point was what distinguished my account of morality from the standard utilitarian account, I was very pleased by its success in persuading the children not to press the doctors to give their father morphine but to wait out the three or four days that their father would live without food and fluids.

When I left them, they seemed completely reconciled to what was happening. They were pleased to know that the stopping of food and fluids meant that they no longer had an indefinite amount of time to wait, and they were prepared to accept my philosophical defense of the difference between active and passive euthanasia and not to press for active euthanasia. I was pleased with the way things had turned out. We had had a satisfying conversation, in which I had provided them with new relevant information about the stopping of food and fluids and with a clear account of the moral relevance of the distinction between active and passive euthanasia. The son and daughter had not merely grudgingly accepted what I had to say, simply regarding me as the final authority sent to enforce the doctor's point of view. They seemed to me to have understood what I was saying and to have genuinely changed their minds about the moral acceptability of pressuring the doctors and nurses to give morphine to their father.

To my great surprise this unhurried philosophical conversation took only forty-five minutes, for it was only 11:45 A.M. when I returned to the nurses' station. I left a message for the resident that the children now understood that the stopping of food and fluids would result in their father's death in less than a week and that they would no longer press for morphine to be given. The resident never called back to find out any more about the case. I was somewhat upset because not only was my distinction between active and passive euthanasia shown to be of practical value, but my moral theory had also been shown to have some significant use, and I wanted to tell this to someone.

Postscript

At the next monthly meeting of the ethics committee I presented an account of my consultation. This is standard procedure for consultations. As I was proceeding, I noticed that a new member of the committee, a member of the Department of Community and Family Medicine, seemed to be enjoying my account more than usual. After I finished, he told me that he was the family doctor referred to and that he had been in contact with the son and daughter after their father had died. He confirmed that their account of our conversation and its outcome were substantially as I had reported it. However, he had two rather minor corrections. First, their father had not died until the following Tuesday; he had taken ten days rather than a week to die. The children were not upset by this, and they had had no second thoughts about pressing for morphine to be given. It turns out that I was wrong in stating that a week is the normal amount of time that it takes a person to die when they are given no fluids. That is the normal amount of time that it takes to become unconscious, but it often takes ten days to two weeks to die.

The second point was that they were not so persuaded by my distinction between thinking about the kind of policy they would want instituted instead of just the consequences of one particular act. Rather, they were deeply affected by the feelings of the nurse who might be giving the morphine when their father died. They did not want to be responsible for causing that kind of situation.

This is the first of several cases that describe gravely ill or seriously handicapped infants. These cases raise difficult ethical issues. When, if ever, should infants have their life support withdrawn and be allowed to die? And who should make that decision? Should parents have unlimited discretion in deciding whether to allow their infant to die? If their discretion should not be unlimited, what should its limits be? Reasonable, well-intentioned persons disagree, intensely and sometimes bitterly, in their answers to these questions. Not only is there ethical disagreement, there is disagreement about the import of various laws and regulations that address the issue of allowing infants to die. What do these regulations actually say, and how seriously need they be taken? Larry Nelson gives a useful overview of many of these issues.

And the Truth Shall Set You Free: The Case of Baby Boy Cory

Lawrence J. Nelson, Ph.D., J.D.

The Case

TWENTY-SIX and a half weeks into a pregnancy marred only by hyperemesis (severe nausea and vomiting) in the first trimester, Mrs. Smith* experienced pink spotting. She called her obstetrician, who told her to take it easy. When the spotting turned bright red

Larry Nelson is a bioethics consultant and attorney in private practice with offices in Berkeley, California.

*The description of the case of Baby Boy "Cory" was prepared by the real Dr. and Mrs. "Smith" with the author's assistance, and they chose to write it in the third person. It reflects *their* recollection of the thoughts, feelings, and conversations they had at the time these events actually took place in 1988. Larry Nelson is the sole author of the Postscript and the Commentary.

later in the day, she called her obstetrician in tears and was told to come to his office.

While her husband, a pediatrician, and four-year-old daughter waited in the hallway, Mrs. Smith lay on the examining table awaiting her physician's reassurance that all was well. She could not suppress a loud cry when he informed her, "You're definitely going over to Labor and Delivery. You're dilated seven centimeters."

Dr. and Mrs. Smith, their daughter, and the obstetrician walked to the adjacent hospital, the child bubbling with excitement that their baby was coming before the neighbors'. The three adults muttered oaths of disbelief.

As a pediatrician, Dr. Smith was well aware of the long-term problems associated with premature birth, including such neurological deficits as cerebral palsy, mental retardation, seizures, and hearing and vision loss, as well as a host of other problems that could occur during the neonatal period. Having been married to Dr. Smith throughout his medical training, Mrs. Smith had listened to hours of medical students' and residents' discussions on the excesses of the neonatal intensive care unit (NICU). To her, the NICU sounded like a baby torture chamber, and she had always sworn that she would never allow a child of hers to be admitted to one. Her fear that her baby would die was nearly matched by her fear that the baby would not be allowed to die should the time come.

Upon arrival at Labor and Delivery Mrs. Smith undressed, had her vital signs and blood taken, and was fitted with an external fetal monitor. Dr. Smith arranged for a friend to pick up their daughter. When Dr. Smith returned to his wife in the labor room, she asked him several disconnected medical questions, pleaded with him not to let their baby go to the NICU, and interspersed it all with nervous jokes about the loud groaning of the laboring woman in the next room.

A neonatology fellow entered the room and introduced herself to the parents. She knew that Dr. Smith was a pediatrician and seemed to feel awkward because of it. He asked her a question that he later learned had branded him as a "difficult parent" among the hospital staff. The question, based on his knowledge of the likely prognosis for an infant born at 26½ weeks, was simply "Do you have to resuscitate? Can you just give us the baby, let us hold him?" "No, I am sorry." A long pause. "But we will continually reassess the situation as things progress. You can discuss it with the attending."

The attending neonatologist entered the room soon thereafter. The father asked her, too, if he and his wife could simply be given the baby to hold upon its birth. She answered, "No. If the baby is vigorous, we have to resuscitate." Looking at the tracing from the fetal monitor, she added, "And the baby looks vigorous now."

"We'll keep reassessing as things progress," she continued. She went on to give Dr. and Mrs. Smith survival statistics for babies born at twenty-six and twenty-seven weeks at that hospital. In stark contrast to the somber mood that pervaded the room, she spoke optimistically of how frequently such babies did well. Dr. Smith was dubious, but feeling that his job as the father was to be supportive and positive, he concluded that this was not the time for doubt or discussion. Mrs. Smith was in a state of general disbelief. She was supposed to be pregnant for another three months but would shortly give birth.

Mrs. Smith was wheeled on a gurney past the unnatural, uncomfortable hush at the nurses' station into the surreal atmosphere of the delivery room. The lights were set low, and the infant resuscitation table was set up and surrounded by the neonatologist, neonatology fellow, senior pediatrics resident, and pediatric intern. Dr. Smith exchanged uncomfortable greetings with the intern, with whom he had worked in the past. He distracted himself for a while watching these physicians repeatedly squeeze the infant resuscitation bag, noting a small release of anxiety with each inflation, but this lasted only momentarily.

The obstetrician and nurse discussed mundane things and joked with the expectant couple with some success. The fetal monitor clicked continuously. The atmosphere could not have been more charged.

Although Mrs. Smith's cervix had dilated the full ten centimeters necessary to give birth, true labor was never established, even after the obstetrician ruptured the membranes. The labor was very difficult because Mrs. Smith could barely feel contractions. "I think I'm having a contraction." Eyes looked toward the fetal tracing. "Yes, I think so. Bear down . . . push, push, push." The pushing ended in a flood of tears.

"Should I push? I can't feel anything. Is this really happening?"

"You've got to push. Good . . . good. There's the head. Stop pushing now."

Finally, the baby was born and immediately resuscitated by the neonatologists. The baby was stabilized and shown to the parents. Dr. Smith saw his wife instantly become a proud mother. "Oh, look, he's so little. He looks like my mother." He could tell immediately that it didn't really matter how big he was or who he looked like; she had her little boy, and she loved him.

For the next hour, the father shuttled back and forth between the nursery and the postpartum recovery area. He was told little about his son's condition and asked no questions. He found that the huddle of people around the baby's warming bed kept him at a distance. However, he did learn that his son's endotracheal tube became plugged at one point, an event that he knew was a risk factor for hypoxia and subsequent neurological damage. Nevertheless, he thought the baby was doing well, and his ventilator settings were moderate. Everyone was optimistic. The father signed some consent forms and went home for the night.

Mrs. Smith was in bed on the regular obstetrics ward. She tried to eat the vending machine sandwich that a nurse had brought her and felt herself to be the definition of aloneness.

Finally, a nurse's aide thought to ask her if she wanted to see her baby. She was surprised to be allowed to and answered with an emphatic "Yes!" She rode in a wheelchair down the long corridor into what looked to her like the spaceship environment of the NICU.

There he lay, in a clear plastic box, attached to an incomprehensible tangle of tubes and wires, her sweet little baby boy. She had loved him from the moment she had known he existed and was heartbroken by her inability to help him now.

Back in her room, unable to sleep, she called her husband. She told him that she still expected to leave the hospital pregnant the next day, and they began to think of a name for the baby. After hanging up the phone, she took a sedative and finally slept.

Dr. Smith was awakened at 2 A.M. by the phone. "Doctor, this is the nursery. I am sorry to tell you that your son developed a pneumothorax [a leak in his lungs], and we have placed a chest tube. He seems to have tolerated this fairly well. I will call you if anything else happens." He simply said, "Thank you," and hung up. Though he knew that a collapsed lung was a red flag for possible lung and neurological damage, he remained hopeful that everything would be all right.

Mrs. Smith awoke early the next morning, felt her nearly flat stomach, and wondered yet again if she had really given birth the night before. When her husband arrived at the hospital, they went together to the NICU. He did not want to enter when he saw a crowd of staff around the baby's incubator, so they waited at the nursery door. Then he told her that the baby had "blown a pneumothorax."

"Oh, no!" Mrs. Smith cried. "No chest tubes! Please, Adam, I don't want him to have a chest tube."

"It's already in. They had to give him a chest tube."

"Can't we do anything to stop it?"

"No."

When Dr. Smith was a medical student, he had explained to his wife how a chest tube was placed. A small slit was cut in the skin of the chest, and then a tube was punched through the chest wall to let off the collection of air. She knew there was a general reluctance to anesthetize sick preemies, and to her the chest tube was the essence of NICU barbarism.

Mrs. Smith was bewildered by a system that could force her child to stay alive, to be tortured by technology, against her will. She felt that her child's premature birth was a mistake of nature that this sort of human interference could only compound. She knew, in a suddenly palpable way, that there were many who disagreed with her, but she believed that where reasonable people could differ, the feelings of the parents should be held paramount. They were the ones who loved him, who could most clearly see beyond their broad philosophical views to his individual best interests. But fearing there was nothing they could do, and still in a highly charged, unbelieving emotional state, she simply tried to absorb and cope with the situation for the time being.

Dr. Smith realized that he was quite passive during his son's first few days of life and was purposely uninvolved in his treatment because he didn't want to interfere with any medical decisions that would have to be made. He felt that he wanted to be his son's father, not his doctor.

On his first full day of life the baby showed one of the common complications of prematurity, extensive bruising with subsequent hyperbilirubinemia (a high level of bilirubin in the blood), but he was not requiring as much assistance with breathing. The father requested that a head ultrasound be performed on the baby that day. It was performed the following day, and the results came back late in the afternoon. The parents were informed by the attending neonatologist that their son had a Grade III intraventricular hemorrhage, a finding associated with brain damage. Dr. Smith knew that premature babies often had such bleeds. He had been hoping that if his son had a head bleed, it would be a grade I or II, which carries a much smaller chance of the child's being badly brain-damaged. Dr. Smith was devastated; this was what he had feared the most. He was further troubled by the hedging he heard in the attending neonatologist's voice and saw in her demeanor. He was left with the impression that the test results could be worse and wondered whether it really was a Grade III bleed. This doubt haunted him all day and led him to the medical library to review the most recent studies about intraventricular hemorrhages and outcome. What kind of a future did his son have to look forward to?

[Author's note: Much later, Dr. Smith found out from contacts on the medical staff of the hospital in which his son was a patient that the attending neonatologist had not been completely honest with him about the results of the ultrasound scans. One contact told Dr. Smith that he had heard her admit that she knew it was a Grade IV hemorrhage despite telling the parents that it was a Grade III. Dr. Smith obtained further confirmation of this after he saw a copy of a report submitted by the attending neonatologist to a state agency that described the hemorrhage as Grade IV. After learning this, Dr. Smith confronted the physician with the discrepancy. She said first that she had not read the report before it went out and that the discrepancy was a typographical error. Then she said her interpretation of the results was a Grade III, but the hospital radiologist's interpretation was Grade IV. Consult the "Postscript" for further discussion of this subject.]

On Day 2 after birth, the baby had a second pneumothorax and another complication of prematurity, a patent ductus arteriosus (a persistence of part of the fetal blood circulation). On Day 3, more complications: refractory acidosis, hypotension, and severe hyperkalemia. Dr. Smith knew that all of these problems are associated with an increased risk of a poor neurological outcome. On Day 4, another ultrasound of the baby's head was performed. The parents were informed by the attending neonatologist that there was no change in the results, but the father still heard hedging in her otherwise reassuring voice. The parents were puzzled when a nurse on the evening shift told them that she was sorry to hear that their son had a Grade IV head bleed but that adults with such bleeds often do all right.

Mrs. Smith had begun to educate herself during this time on the long-term problems of prematurity that most concerned her husband, but she also read numerous parents' accounts of their experiences with premature babies. For every medical statistic that said virtually all babies like theirs fared poorly, there was a joyful parent who described a one-in-a-million miracle baby with bilateral Grade IV hemorrhages and double shunts for hydrocephalus who was reading by age two.

Taken in conjunction with stories like this, Mrs. Smith started to believe the smiling, upbeat encouragements of the nursery staff. NICU procedures seemed less barbaric as she grew accustomed to chest tubes, CO_2 monitors, endotracheal tubes, and endless heel sticks. She let herself be convinced that an obvious grimace of pain was just her baby's normal wish to cry. She wanted to believe that a modern medical miracle could let her keep her little baby boy.

A new neonatologist took over the baby's care on Day 5. On the same day, Dr. Smith asked a pediatric neurologist who was a friend of his to become involved in the case and help clarify things. She recommended that frequent ultrasound scans of the head be done. Both the neurologist and the father talked to the new attending neonatologist about this, and he reluctantly agreed.

The baby's condition remained largely unchanged on Day 6. The nurses were encouraging and supportive. There was extremely limited contact between the new attending neonatologist and the parents. It seemed to the father that the attending neonatologist was doing his best to avoid both him and his wife. His response to even the most direct questions about the child's condition was a vague listing of the potential outcomes.

On Day 7, on the advice of the neurologist, Dr. Smith took the ultrasound pictures for interpretation to two physicians who practiced at a different hospital. Only one of these physicians was available, and he reported his interpretation of the scans as showing without much doubt a Grade IV hemorrhage, with possible bleeding bilaterally and cystic lesions, though it was too early to determine this. He added that he was not as experienced at interpreting such scans as the other physician and urged the father to return the following day for her review of the scans.

On Day 8, Dr. Smith returned for the interpretation of the head scans by the second physician. She confirmed that it was a Grade IV hemorrhage and stated: "Based on my experience but not on any studies, it is very probable that your son will have multiple and severe neurological deficits. I can say with 100 percent certainty that he will not be normal neurologically. On a scale of one to ten, with ten being the worst, I would call this a six, or maybe a seven or eight." She did not, however, quantify what she meant by "very probable."

After hearing this, the father was certain that his son's life support should be terminated. His thinking about the situation had clarified: it would be an acceptable outcome if his son were to be somewhat mentally retarded or have some kind of motor problem, but multiple and severe neurological problems like cerebral palsy, seizures, and profound mental retardation was an unacceptable outcome. At this point, he had little doubt that termination of further medical treatment was in his *son's* best interest. He thought: "For me, there are no other considerations such as what this will do to my family or what his care might cost. It is my responsibility to see that *he* not be made to endure a life characterized by pain, suffering, rejection, and failure, an existence best described as lying somewhere between pity and tolerance. Though he put no exact number on his son's chances to be severely brain-damaged, he knew that the chances were simply too high not to do something about them.

Dr. Smith called his wife at the NICU and asked her to pick him up so that they could return to the hospital together. She had been enjoying a rare moment of pleasure with her sick newborn. She read and sang to him, watching his facial muscles relax and his pulse and blood pressure settings on the monitor go down in response to the sound of her voice. She felt less helpless and more hopeful than she had since his birth, and she resented her husband's intrusive demand, which he refused to explain over the telephone, that she pick him up immediately.

But she went, and when he got into the car she growled at him, "Don't ever do that to me again. For the first time, I was really enjoying my baby."

Her husband was talking over her, neither listening to the other, when finally he shouted, "He's going to be a vegetable!"

"No! No! Don't say that!"

"I have to. It's true. Two experts in the field just told me."

"Oh, my God . . ."

After her angry shouts had dissolved into tears, then silence, and his into an imperative speech on how strong she would have to be, they drove back to the hospital. On the way, he explained that he could no longer say that everything was going to be all right.

When they arrived at the hospital, the mother went to visit her son, and the father went to find the attending neonatologist. He was taken aback by Dr. Smith's request that treatment be discontinued but listened empathetically and made no direct response other than to say that he was ambivalent. After he heard the interpretation of the scans by the outside physician, he said he wanted to hear the interpretation directly from the physician who made it. The father then tried to reach this physician, but she had left her office for the day to begin a month's vacation out of the country. He then called his friend, the neurologist, and asked for her help. Things were left hanging that day. Dr. Smith had no doubts about what he was asking to have done. Mrs. Smith, on the other hand, was in a state of intense emotional turmoil and confusion. Lacking her husband's firm conviction, she stayed in the background, observed her baby, and tried to learn as much as she could and sort out her own feelings.

On the morning of the next day (Day 9), the attending neonatologist called Dr. Smith at his home. Dr. Smith asked the physician what he intended to do, whether he would discontinue support. After several minutes of listening to him equivocate, Dr. Smith yelled, "Tell me what the hell you are going to do. Give me a straight answer." The neonatologist said that he could not and would not discontinue support.

The parents went to the hospital again. Mrs. Smith visited the baby while the father tried to meet with the neonatologist. He plainly didn't want to talk to Dr. Smith and made him wait over an hour before agreeing to talk to him. Dr. Smith first asked him why he wouldn't discontinue support.

"There is always the possibility that the child could have a chance for a reasonable life."

"What's a reasonable life?" asked the father.

"Independent living."

"Would you take responsibility for this child?"

"In a sense, I do."

The father continued. "Would you take him home? Help support his special needs, school, training? Would you secure him a future after we were gone? Would you be there to help him understand, if in fact he could understand? Would you explain to my daughter why her life was so drastically changed?" At this point, the father lost control of himself and broke down sobbing.

The neonatologist responded, "No, that is not my responsibility. Life is not fair. That's just the way it is."

"Don't we as parents have any rights, any say in this at all?"

"Well, you can always take him to another nursery, but I doubt that any nursery would take him. You can move him if you like."

Just then, the neurologist who had been involved in the case appeared. She had been asked by the attending neonatologist to examine the baby, even though she had told him that a physical exam would show little in such a young child. However, she had the opportunity to speak to the outside physician who had interpreted the ultrasound scans before she left on vacation.

Shortly thereafter, there was another meeting among the neurologist, the father, the attending neonatologist, and a colleague of the family's private pediatrician (who had visited the baby every day and written a short note in the chart but otherwise had played no role in the child's care). The neurologist confirmed the interpretation of the scans the father had received on Days 7 and 8. The neonatologist still wanted more information. After some further discussion, all agreed that a CT scan should be done to clarify the extent of the brain damage.

The father returned home. Sensing that the neonatologist was not going to honor the request to discontinue treatment, he began making calls to find someone who might help him and his wife contend with this situation. One of his thoughts during this time was to ask the attending neonatologist if he would be willing to sign a letter of intent to provide direct financial and social support for his child in order to make this responsibility more than a theoretical construct.

Some two hours after returning home, he received a call from the neonatologist, who said that he did not believe that the baby was stable enough for a CT scan. He added, "It doesn't matter anyway. The results of the CT scan won't change my decision. The only time I would consider withdrawing support would be if your son developed severe necrotizing enterocolitis [NEC] and perforated his bowel. Then I might not send him to the operating room."

As the father knew that the hospital had an ethics committee and that he disagreed with the neonatologist ethically, he then asked the neonatologist whether a meeting of the ethics committee could be convened to discuss the case. He replied, "There is no need. We have a policy against discontinuing life support. The decision is not the committee's to make but mine as the attending physician." The conversation ended, and the ethics committee was never consulted. There had been no mention of such a policy any time prior to this.

Dr. Smith called the private pediatrician who attended the conference earlier in the day. He said he found the situation disturbing but was not inclined to take any action. Dr. Smith felt that he had no recourse within the medical community to help him deal with the situation and after some hesitation decided to make contact with an ethicist/attorney (L. Nelson) whose name he had obtained earlier in the day after making numerous phone calls. Dr. Smith felt the matter was quite urgent, as his son might soon improve to the point where he could breathe on his own, and this would complicate the issue of forgoing treatment.

By this time, Mrs. Smith's own feelings were becoming clearer. After days of ruthless soul-searching, she was somewhat able to separate hope from reality and her own interests from those of her child. For her own sake, she wanted him to live. She wanted to hold him, to cuddle him, to watch him grow. She wanted to see his little baby smiles and hear his little baby sounds. She knew that these desires fed her hopes that he could be only slightly handicapped or be a happy child despite severe handicaps. She agonized over her fear that in attempting to save him from a living hell, they might also be depriving him of living joy.

But as much as she hoped that he could be okay, she knew that objectively this was unlikely. Although no expert could tell them for sure what their child's ultimate condition would be, the risks for cerebral palsy and serious mental retardation were very high. She did not feel that she had the right to expose her child to these risks.

In addition, when the neonatologist mentioned that he might treat the baby for severe NEC, she was horrified. It seemed to her that they wanted to push him to the very limits of pain before allowing him the respite of death. She was reminded of how rocky his neonatal course could still be, and she regained her original pure impulse to spare him from the suffering imposed by neonatal technology. Forcing him to endure a painful infancy to face the sort of life that likely awaited him was simply wrong. Still, she felt helpless against the stone wall of hospital policy, and she admired her husband's bravery and diligence in the search for ways to save their child.

Dr. Smith called Mr. Nelson late in the afternoon of Day 9 and explained the situation. Mr. Nelson assured him that he and his wife did indeed have control over the medical care their son would receive, though not unlimited control. In any event, the attending neonatologist was simply wrong, both ethically and legally, in asserting that they had no say whatsoever in determining their child's medical fate. He explained that the courts in California and around the country had decided very few cases involving the termination of treatment of a newborn. A California statute, part of the child abuse laws, did set forth a general standard: an "informed and appropriate medical decision" made by a parent in consultation with a physician who had actually examined the child was not medical neglect. He noted that there was no statutory definition of an "informed and appropriate medical decision" and that no appellate court had interpreted this statute in a published decision.

Mr. Nelson also discussed the federal law pertaining to the medical treatment of seriously ill and disabled infants, the Child Abuse Amendments of 1984. He informed the father that the State of California had not yet implemented this law, although compliance should have occurred by October 1985, and that, in his opinion, this law was not controlling in his son's case. He added that there was disagreement among some experts about his position and that this law was aimed directly at the type of case this child presented: a non-terminally ill infant with a medical condition that would potentially leave him with serious neurological disabilities. He mentioned that, based on his knowledge of the hospital that was caring for the child, it was very likely that the physicians involved were motivated by legal concerns instilled by the hospital's legal counsel, who usually took a rigid position against forgoing treatment.

He also observed that there was still a great deal of controversy among ethicists about the propriety of forgoing treatment of seriously ill and handicapped infants. He observed that although there was significant agreement on the applicability of the "best interests of the child" standard, agreement was lacking as to the precise meaning of this standard. Dr. Smith replied that he strongly believed discontinuing treatment was in his son's best interests, as it would be wrong to impose on him an existence characterized by suffering and by living in a society that would pay only the most superficial lip service to him and his great needs. Mr. Nelson told the father that, all things considered, he personally judged his and his wife's decision to be right on the edge of ethical and legal permissibility. He emphasized that many would disagree with their decision and that he was by no means confident that a court would uphold their decision if challenged directly. Dr. Smith said that he understood this, but he still thought forgoing treatment was the right thing for his son.

Mr. Nelson recommended that they try to have the child transferred to another intensive care nursery where the staff might be more open to the parents' point of view, as this would probably be the best way to achieve their end while avoiding a direct confrontation with the physicians and hospital currently treating their son. He added that the present providers would be hard-pressed to object to a transfer to an appropriate institution willing to accept medical responsibility. Dr. Smith and Mr. Nelson agreed to work together on effectuating a transfer within a few days, and Mr. Nelson agreed to represent the parents as an attorney (rather than as a consulting ethicist) as this would afford their relationship the confidentiality of the attorney-client privilege. As Mr. Nelson was leaving town for a few days, they agreed to talk again when he returned. After this conversation, Dr. Smith felt that there was at least some basis for discussion of what he sought.

The following day (Day 10), Dr. Smith spoke to the pediatric neurologist. She reported that she had great difficulty in getting the attending neonatologist to talk to her about the results of the CT scan that she thought had been performed. Only by means of vociferous insistence was she able to talk to him and discover that the CT scan had not been done because the child purportedly was too unstable. She thought that this explanation was fabricated, and she recommended that the baby be transferred elsewhere where the physicians would behave in a more reasonable manner. Dr. Smith contacted a neonatologist at another hospital, who agreed to accept the transfer and who indicated a willingness to consider the parents' wishes after examining the situation. Dr. Smith called the attending neonatologist, who said that a transfer was fine with him. The neonatologist left him with the distinct impression that he was really happy about the prospect of being rid of the case. A few hours later the baby was transferred. That evening, the child had several tonic/clonic seizures, another poor neurological prognostic sign.

At this point, the father felt that although he did want support withdrawn because he was convinced that it was in his son's best interests to do so, this was not the primary reason for the transfer. He felt that they (though he much more so than his wife) were in conflict with the neonatologist, who had always and quite obviously avoided both of them when they were in the nursery. He also felt that the neonatologist was uncomfortable in talking to them even before the issue of withdrawing support had been raised. Worst of all, the neonatologist had not been honest. Instead of telling the parents his own policy or that of the hospital right from the start, he had said nothing. In response to specific questions from the father about what might be done if certain things were to occur, the neonatologist had said that the situation would surely be reassessed in that event. In fact, though, there could be no reassessment. Dr. Smith thought: The doors were closed to my son from the beginning. I thought that the question of withdrawal of support was open and at least deserving of discussion. There would obviously be none of that here.

The next day (Day 11 after birth) a CT scan was performed at the second hospital without incident, and the neonatologists reviewed the case in detail. A long and involved discussion then occurred among the new attending neonatologist, the neonatology fellow, the neurologist who had been involved in the case all along, and the parents. The providers offered the parents their interpretation of the imaging studies that had been done: although the data were not exact and they could not predict the baby's neurological outcome with any certainty, they believed he had suffered neurological damage that could range from mild to major. They acknowledged that medical technology had created this kind of situation and that it was a hard choice for all involved. They offered the parents the options of maintaining the status quo, of not resuscitating the child in the event of a cardiac arrest, or of withdrawing ventilatory support. The risks and complications of each were explained, including the "risk" that he would continue to breathe on his own off the ventilator. They also mentioned that the parents were not being offered special treatment because the father was a physician; any parent in this situation would be offered the same options. The physicians also made clear that they would not give the child a large dose of sedative or morphine to hasten his death.

The parents chose to withdraw support. The Smiths were not prepared for the outpouring of support they received for their decision to take their baby off the ventilator, especially from the pediatricians. Many doctors, nurses, and other hospital personnel went out of their way to assure the Smiths that they had "done the right thing." This response led the parents to conclude that even among those with direct daily involvement in children's health care, there is no monolithic support for a "life at any cost" approach to neonatology. For Mrs. Smith, who didn't know if she would ever fully resolve the issues surrounding her son's birth and death, these assurances brought an immense sense of relief. The decision to let their baby go, which would have involved the simple pain of losing a baby if it could have been made at his birth, had been nearly unendurable once he had lived eleven days. It was a decision that no parent should ever have to make, and yet it was a decision that only a parent, with the advice and support of caring physicians, could make.

After he was removed from the ventilator, the mother cradled her son and took many pictures of him. The parents had spent three hours with the baby when he died quietly in their arms. The father recalled later that it was at this time "that we got to know and say good-bye to our son."

Postscript

Some nine months after these events took place, the parents and I (LJN) obtained their son's medical records. A review of them yielded some interesting information.

First, the original attending neonatologist's off-service summary
(Day 4) described the intraventricular hemorrhage as Grade IV. One of
her progress notes (Day 3) called it a "Grade III–IV" bleed. The report
of the radiologist who interpreted the first head ultrasound (Day 2)
characterized the hemorrhage as "Grade III$^1/_2$" but noted that it would
be a Grade IV if "the right periventricular echogenicity is due to hemorrhage, not ischemia." Given the location of the brain damage, it is
doubtful whether this distinction makes any difference in the child's
prognosis. As it is not standard practice for physicians to use the term
"III$^1/_2$" to describe the severity of an intraventricular hemorrhage in a
newborn, its use can probably best be attributed to waffling on the part
of the interpreter. One pediatric neurologist I consulted called this term
"slippery, very slippery." All progress notes (other than the one mentioned above from Day 3) written by residents or other physicians
called the hemorrhage Grade IV.

Second, only two of the many nursing notes mention the existence of
an intraventricular hemorrhage. One (Day 8) called it a Grade II or III.
The other (Day 7) addressed the father's feelings about his son's neurological condition: "Dad very concerned about babe's head bleed and
outcome." No nursing note referred to the parents' request to discontinue treatment or to any reason for the baby's transfer to another
hospital.

Third, a progress note written by the second attending neonatologist
at an undisclosed time on Day 9 (the day after the parents first stated
they wanted treatment discontinued and the day he disclosed the "policy" against withdrawing life support), made no mention of the parents' wishes or the policy. The note observed that the child "neurologically remains active with surprisingly normal exam," that the
outside physician who first reviewed the sonogram "felt that the blood
[in the right side of the brain] is suggestive of Grade IV hemorrhage,"
and that "we are continuing to have discussions with the parents about
the implications of these findings."

The same neonatologist's progress note on Day 10, the date of the
baby's transfer to the other hospital, referred to "continuing discussions with the father concerning the child's prognosis and the appropriateness of the level of support [of] the child in light of his guarded
neurological prognosis" and simply stated that "the father transferred
the child to [another hospital] for further therapy." No reason for the
transfer was offered.

Finally, the following is an excerpt from a report written by a physician at the second hospital shortly after Cory's death. "Several hours after admission . . . there were generalized tonic-clonic seizures noted. The infant was given 10 mg/kg phenobarbital, and there was no recurrence of the seizures. A CT scan was performed and this confirmed the diagnosis [of intraventricular hemorrhage] . . . . The previous sonograms and CT scan and the infant's clinical condition were discussed with the Pediatric Neurology attending staff. The long term prognosis for this infant at 27 weeks gestation with a grade IV [intraventricular hemorrhage] and generalized seizures was discussed with the parents. The high probability of severe long term neurological morbidity was discussed. At the parents' request mechanical ventilation was discontinued and the infant expired shortly thereafter."

Commentary

In my work as a bioethics consultant, I am usually asked to become involved in a clinical case by a physician, nurse, administrator, or hospital ethics committee. Thus, those who are providing health care to a particular patient are the ones who usually want me to help them struggle with an ethical dilemma or question. Occasionally, I am contacted by parents or family members of patients who want to consult with me.

For example, I have been consulted by the parents of a boy who was dying of irreversible liver disease in a state-operated institution for the developmentally disabled. They asked me if anything could be done to allow their son to die peacefully rather than to be transported frequently to an acute-care hospital where, in unfamiliar surroundings, he received painful treatment that could not cure him but did prolong his dying. When they had asked the institution's medical director if their son could be kept there and allowed to die comfortably in what had become his home rather than in a hospital, they were told they would be murderers to do such a thing. More recently, I was contacted by Dr. Smith, whose newborn son Cory lay in an intensive care nursery suffering from the effects of prematurity and a serious hemorrhage inside his head.

Parents' Role in Clinical Decision Making

In this case, the physicians caring for Cory let the parents know, both directly and indirectly, that their son's medical fate was outside their control. They were not permitted to assume an active role in making decisions about the medial treatment Cory would or would not receive. Rather, the parents were to be informed about the physician's treatment decisions and apparently expected to endorse them without question. The second attending neonatologist's assumption of unilateral control over treatment decisions is best seen in his words to the father on Day 9: "The *only* time *I* would consider withdrawing support would be if your son developed severe necrotizing enterocolitis and perforated his bowel. Then *I might not send* him to the operating room" (emphasis added). In this physician's eyes, the child's medical fate was to be determined by his orders much as a soldier's fate would be determined by the orders of his commanding officer.

Despite many calls from ethicists and others for joint decision making between physicians and parents about a child's medical care, parents not infrequently are disenfranchised from participation in determining the course of their child's care, particularly if the child is critically ill and in an intensive care unit. Such disenfranchisement can occur despite the fact that the parents are well educated or articulate individuals (as were Dr. and Mrs. Smith) who understand their child's medical situation quite well. If it was very hard for a physician like Dr. Smith (and a pediatrician to boot) to deal with the medical establishment, then it must be incalculably harder for a nonphysician, a less-educated person, or a less doggedly determined person to do so. Any parents who are trying to cope with the emotional upheaval caused by the birth of a very sick child are in a poor position to assert their right to be involved in their child's medical care in the face of physician opposition.

There are a number of reasons for this phenomenon. First, some physicians simply reject the notion of sharing decision-making authority with the parents and consider themselves solely responsible and best qualified for this task. This view is not limited to crusty, paternalistic pediatricians of the "old school." Both neonatologists involved in Cory's case were young and recently trained in modern medical centers.

Second, many physicians rather uncritically assume that parents of seriously ill newborns are too overwhelmed by anxiety, grief, guilt, and shock to make "good" decisions about their child's care. Third, neonatologists often have great difficulty contending with the uncertainty inherent in their diagnoses and prognoses of very ill newborns, much less disclosing and explaining this uncertainty to worried parents.

Hence, they find it easier to make authoritative and optimistic pro-
nouncements about the child's care that camouflages this uncertainty.
Last, and by no means least, neonatologists are frequently befuddled
by the ethical and legal controversy that swirls around the question of
forgoing treatment of critically ill or handicapped newborns. Consequently, they have serious trouble identifying the ethical and legal
boundaries of medical and parental discretion in deciding to allow an
infant to die. Ignoring parental requests to forgo treatment or not even
considering forgoing treatment eliminates the need to find these elusive boundaries.

When Dr. Smith initially contacted me, the first question he wanted
answered was who had the authority to make medical treatment decisions for his son. Were these physicians right? Did he and his wife have
any say in Cory's medical care? The tone of his voice made clear that he
was greatly distressed by the thought that he had no control over the
outcome of his child's care. I tried to reassure him as best I could that
the physicians were not right in taking unilateral control over Cory's
medical treatment.

Parents do have the authority to give or withhold their consent to
medical treatment of their child and have rather broad discretion in
exercising this authority, though it is subject to imperfectly defined and
understood ethical and legal limits. As a report of the President's Commission for the Study of Ethical Problems in Medicine stated: "There is
a presumption, strong but rebuttable, that parents are the appropriate
decision-makers for their infants. Traditional law concerning the family, buttressed by the emerging constitutional right of privacy, protects
a substantial range of discretion for parents." The U.S. Supreme Court
has also referred with approval to a summary of the law in this regard
prepared by the federal secretary of health and human services: "The
decision to provide or withhold medically indicated treatment is, except in highly unusual circumstances, made by the parents or legal
guardian" (*Bowen v. American Hospital Assn.*, 106 S.Ct. 2101, 1986).

Sound ethical values undergird this legal policy. A child does, after
all, belong to his or her parents—but not like an object that is theirs to
use, abuse, destroy, or discard. The child is their flesh and blood, their
responsibility. The child is in a human family they have created. Parents have natural bonds of affection for and loyalty to that child that no
one else has to quite the same extent. Of course, not all parents treat
their children with love and loyalty. However, in the absence of compelling evidence to the contrary, we assume that the parents are the best

people to raise a child—or at a minimum, the least detrimental care-takers.[1]

Parents are also the ones who have to live with the child after all is said and done. The physicians, nurses, social workers, lawyers, or judges who may get involved do not have to live with the child and care for him or her every day, to experience the outcome of what may be only partially effective medical technology, and to witness and bear responsibility for how the child fares in this far from sympathetic and trouble-free world. This is *not* to say parents should have complete control over their child's destiny, but only that they should have relatively broad discretion in making choices about their own child's health care. And these choices need not receive unanimous approval from the rest of us, though they should be reasonable, acceptable, tolerable.

Finally, we should be reluctant to second-guess parents too readily because there is no assurance that strangers removed from the actual circumstances, with no bonds of parental love or loyalty, will make a better decision than the parents will. In an imperfect world, parents will usually, though by no means always, be the best people to make important decisions about their child's life.

In sum, it is paternalistic, presumptuous, and wrong—both ethically and legally—for physicians to tell parents outright, to imply, or to act as if they have no authority over their children's medical care. Consequently, the central issue between the physicians and Cory's parents should not have been whether the latter had any control over the course of their son's medical care, but rather whether their request to discontinue life support was beyond the limits of their discretion as parents and could rightly be characterized as unacceptable medical neglect. Individual neonatologists, nurses, ethicists, clergy, parents, and others are struggling with this issue, as is a society that has laws forbidding parents from medically neglecting a child. Cory's physicians and his parents never even mentioned this issue, much less discussed it openly and honestly.

To be sure, there will be cases in which the functional ability of the parents to participate meaningfully and responsibly in the decision-making process about their child's clinical care is so compromised by the effects of substance abuse (alcohol, drugs, etc.), grief, intrafamily disagreements, or mental illness that clinicians may have to proceed on their own, at least for a time. But this case was definitely not in that category. These parents were ready, willing, and manifestly able to participate in making decisions about their child's care but were denied this burdensome but necessary responsibility.

The Limits of Parental Discretion in Deciding to Forgo Treatment

I struggled with identifying the limits of parental discretion in this case because I knew I could not in good conscience advise or represent the parents effectively if I honestly thought they had clearly crossed the line and made an unacceptable decision about Cory's care. As a lawyer and a citizen, I believe that even those I personally view as "in the wrong" (e.g., an indisputably guilty criminal defendant or a neo-Nazi who wants to exercise free but despicable speech in public) deserve legal representation. But as an individual, I knew I could not advocate a point of view that I had concluded was plainly unethical and harmful to a child.

Interestingly, my wife was about fourteen weeks pregnant at the time Dr. Smith consulted me, and his story spurred me to think long and hard about what I might do if my child were like Cory. In truth, I did not know what I would do if it were my child, but I did not believe then (nor do I now) that these parents had made a patently unreasonable and unacceptable decision in light of their child's serious prematurity and probably severe neurological damage. Yet I still had my doubts.

The boundaries of parental discretion in cases involving critically ill, premature, severely asphyxiated, or seriously neurologically compromised newborns are not readily identifiable, whether one utilizes a general ethical standard (e.g., "the best interests of the child") or a legal standard like the one in California (viz., "an informed and appropriate medical decision" by parents is not medical neglect). The practical meaning of such standards will not be ascertained in the abstract but only amid the circumstances of individual cases. Unfortunately, not enough discussion among neonatologists, ethicists, parents, and others is occurring around the facts and circumstances of individual cases with the express intent of utilizing the case to identify both the ethically relevant features and how we should sift through these features to arrive at a clinically responsible decision about a child's fate. Put differently, we need to reflect on individual cases to find out why we think a certain decision is or is not within the range of reasonable and acceptable parental discretion, even though all may not agree with such a decision or make the same decision themselves in similar circumstances.

In general, I believe that a variety of factors should be considered in cases where forgoing further treatment of a seriously ill newborn is being contemplated by some involved person, though *no one* single factor is determinative of an ethically acceptable outcome.

1. *The child's diagnosis and chances for survival.* As a general matter, it is neither medically nor ethically indicated to prolong the dying of any patient.

2. *The child's prognosis for neurological and physical functioning, both with and without treatment.* Parents and clinicians are rightly concerned about what a child's functional abilities will be if he or she survives. Even very ill patients sometimes survive unexpectedly after treatment has been withheld or withdrawn, and both clinicians and parents should be prepared for this and for the fact that forgoing treatment may make such a child worse than he or she would have been with treatment. Although prognostication is fraught with uncertainty, physicians must still do it in order to give parents a realistic, if imperfect, view of what medicine can and cannot do for their child.

3. *The treatment benefits and burdens to the child.* No one should be surprised by the notion that neonatal medicine does not offer only benign treatments to newborns. For example, the medically necessary use of a mechanical ventilator to breathe for a baby can cause irreparable lung damage. Whether NICU care in any given case rises to the level of "barbarism" (as it did in Mrs. Smith's eyes) is an open question: it can do much good for babies and their families, though it can also do harm.

4. *The effect of the child's clinical situation on his or her family.* A child exists in the social context of a family—mother, father, siblings, grandparents—and for the most part, is best left within that family to live and perhaps, sometimes, to die.[2] Long-drawn-out NICU care for a newborn can cause marriages to crack and other children to be neglected by their parents; it can bring out dormant family pathology and lead parents to regress in their ability to cope maturely with their situation. This is *not* to say that a severely ill child should be allowed to die simply because his care will be burdensome, even positively harmful, to his parents, siblings, other family members, or society in general. But such burden and harm to others is not irrelevant to the process of ethical decision making.

5. *The professional and ethical integrity of the NICU staff.* As was mentioned earlier, decisions about a child's medical care should be made jointly between the parents and responsible clinicians. As neonatal

medicine progresses, clinicians develop their own views about what a "good" outcome is, and they can differ from parents' views. Clinicians also have their own ethical values and their own view of their ethical obligations toward patients. This has to be taken into account when decisions are being made about forgoing life-sustaining treatment. In this case, however, it would be odd for the physicians to defend their actions using this rationale given that much of their deceptive and presumptuous behavior reflects so poorly on their professional ethics.

6. *The best interests of the infant.* One commentator, Howard Brody, has called this popular standard "incoherent or inadequate."[3] Another commentator, William Bartholome, has noted that it "does not function well when interpreted as an objective and substantive criteria [sic] for analysis of the *ethical* aspects of a problem in medical ethics. Instead, it has value as a 'conceptual lens'—as a device that assists us in seeing what is at stake in the problem and that directs and focuses the decisionmaking process."[4] He contends that "the best interests of the child" means that the proposed course of medical care "should be undertaken in pursuit of the best interests of the child, and the reasons offered in support should reflect a primary focus on and commitment to the child. Those involved in the decision should see themselves as obligated to protect the child and his or her interests."

My application of the factors outlined above to Cory's case did not lead me to any obvious or inevitable conclusion about the ethical propriety of the parents' wishes. Cory was not irretrievably on his way toward death when I was involved in his case. Nevertheless, the complications of prematurity from which Cory suffered had significantly compromised his chances for survival. Interestingly, one commentator on the ethics of newborn care has stated that 90 percent of newborns with a Grade IV intraventricular hemorrhage die, and the survivors often end up with mental retardation and blindness.[5] Moreover, Cory could die after going through a long stay in the NICU during which he probably would have suffered a great deal from the needlesticks, prodding, tubes, bright lights, medications, and diagnostic procedures necessary to treat him. Yet this very treatment could also save him, and there is no reliable way to predict if he would be one of those who would not survive.

The ethical relevance of the neurological damage Cory probably had suffered is harder and more controversial to assess. Less serious neurological damage could cause the child to have only mild tremors of the limbs and mild mental retardation or learning disabilities. More serious damage could lead to severe cerebral palsy that might leave the child unable to move his limbs and cause severe or profound mental retardation, blindness, and/or deafness, disabling seizure activity, and a shortened life span.

I personally reject both extreme views about the ethical relevance of neurological damage: either that it is immaterial to the justification of forgoing life-sustaining treatment or that it alone is sufficient justification. The former position focuses solely on the child's ability to survive and wrongly excludes from consideration (1) the burdensomeness of the treatment itself for the child; (2) the fact that some neurological damage can be so devastating that a loving parent can conclude he or she lacks (to use Mrs. Smith's words) "the right to expose her child to these risks"; and (3) the not unreasonable belief of some that achieving a person's mere physical survival is just not enough benefit, either humanly or medically speaking, to justify continued treatment. In short, a child's actual or projected quality of life is relevant to decisions about forgoing treatment.

On the other hand, the presence of some neurological or intellectual deficit—that is, some diminishment of the ability to live a "normal" life, is not in itself a sufficiently compelling reason to allow a child to die who otherwise could live with reasonable medical treatment. Consequently, I disagree with the decision of the parents and the Indiana state courts in the original 1983 Baby Doe case to permit a newborn with Down's syndrome (and hence some undeterminable degree of mental retardation) to die without receiving lifesaving surgery to correct a defect that prevented him from taking food or fluid by mouth. In this regard, we also have to be aware that discriminatory attitudes toward the handicapped can influence treatment decisions in an untoward manner. Being handicapped is not necessarily to be doomed to a life not worth living.

I concluded that Cory's parents had not wrongly (and certainly not maliciously) determined that the future their son faced as a result of his medical problems was bleak: he was facing a substantial (and, in their minds, overwhelming) risk that his intellectual and motor abilities would be severely limited. I also concluded that I could not honestly say that their decision was inconsistent with their son's best interests. My judgment about this factor was reinforced by the fact that Cory had a substantial chance of dying no matter what happened. My judgment here was also influenced by the parents' assessment of the relative burdens and benefits of further treatment. They saw their child enduring a great deal in the NICU (and anticipated that he might be required to endure a great deal more in the future), yet they could not see compensating benefits resulting for him.

The parents were not focusing on how Cory's care would burden them or their daughter or how he might complicate their lives with his extensive needs should he survive. Nonetheless, given the strength of their feelings about the suffering that can be caused by aggressive medical treatment in the NICU and by severe functional impairments, I think they knew they would be deeply affected, even devastated, if Cory lived on in a severely impaired or vegetative state and they had not done their best to spare him from such a fate. This was especially true for Dr. Smith, who himself had been born prematurely and had suffered from some resulting mild disabilities. He knew on a personal and elemental level about living with suffering, rejection, and failure, and he knew that his son would probably endure much, much worse than he had faced. I believe he found it simply impossible to leave his son to this fate.

I had to tell Dr. Smith that in the last analysis, I thought that his and his wife's decision was very near the edge of permissibility, that many people would not agree with their decision, and that some might try to prevent them from implementing their decision, including invocation of the legal system. After all, the child was not terminally ill at that point and had a small chance to be free of severe neurological disability. Even if he were to have severe brain damage, that is not necessarily sufficient reason to terminate life-sustaining treatment. The father told me he understood all of this, but his decision remained unchanged.

The Policy against Discontinuing Life Support

The neonatologists did not reveal the existence of a "policy" against discontinuing life support until the day after the parents first requested that treatment be discontinued. When the policy did suddenly appear, it was never explained or justified. Was it a formal, written policy of the hospital? Or was it informal, unwritten, and used on an ad hoc basis as a particular physician wished? Was it a policy of the hospital's organized medical staff or of the neonatologists? What were the reasons for it? Were they ethical, legal, personal, or religious in nature? Did it apply in all cases? Did all neonatologists interpret it in the same way? Did they all agree with it? None of these questions was answered, though the parents surely did not think of asking all of them either. In any event, the attending neonatologist announced this policy to the father over the telephone somewhat like God giving Moses the Ten Commandments, although God at least did it in person. These are the rules. End of discussion.

I was convinced that legal concerns were at the very least lurking barely beneath the surface of this amorphous "policy" and probably were its foundation. Although I had no direct experience with the neonatologists at this particular hospital or firsthand knowledge of their attitudes about forgoing treatment, I was personally acquainted with an ethicist who had dealt with them and who was quite familiar with the hospital generally. He had told me that the neonatologists were fearful about the legal implications of forgoing treatment and therefore were reluctant to do so even at the insistence of the parents in what many would consider to be appropriate cases. I had also heard that the hospital's ethics committee had been floundering partly because the hospital's lawyers seemingly always had the last word on what could and could not be done. I was also acquainted with the lawyers who acted as the hospital's legal counsel in matters like this and knew that they routinely took what I considered to be an extremely conservative position, namely, physicians were legally compelled by the so-called Baby Doe law to treat all infants, with the exception of those who were imminently and inevitably dying.

As I have discussed in more detail elsewhere,[6] the Baby Doe law (actually, the Child Abuse Amendments of 1984) has been imbued with a significance and power entirely out of proportion to what it deserves legally or practically. This is so primarily because of the efforts of the Reagan administration and secondarily because of physicians' dislike and fear of entanglement in the legal system. The gap between the law's image in the minds of many involved in the care of newborns and its reality is wide indeed. In addition, it is becoming apparent that the Baby Doe law has significantly affected the medical care of handicapped and severely ill newborns, mostly in an untoward fashion.[7] Perhaps the most invidious effect of the law is how it seems to have replaced compassionate and careful attention to the best interests of disabled and severely ill newborns with preoccupation about abstract legal formulas, political concerns, and fears of remote possibilities of legal liability. In any event, the Baby Doe law had not been implemented in California at the time Cory was born and has not been as of the writing of this chapter.

Although the law regarding the limits of parental discretion in deciding to forgo life-sustaining treatment for a child is vague and difficult to assess, I do not believe that it absolutely precludes consideration of withdrawing treatment in a case like Cory's. However, I must hasten to add that it is by no means clear that any given trial court judge or appellate panel of judges in California would have permitted the Smiths' wishes to prevail if their decision had been directly challenged in court. Lawyers often find it no easier to predict the legal future and a client's chances of winning in court than physicians do when they try to prognosticate about a patient's medical future and chances of surviving. If I had been forced to give Dr. Smith a prediction, I would have told him that I would consider his chances of having a judge agree with the decision to forgo further treatment probably to be no better than fifty-fifty and perhaps less if he were unable to get other physicians to testify about the medical and ethical acceptability of what he proposed. My explanation for this: (1) the courts are not familiar with these cases and so will tend to rule cautiously; and (2) as usual, the law is behind the professional and ethical thinking on this subject. For this and other reasons, such as my desire to spare the parents (and myself) the publicity that would inevitably surround any court proceeding and my belief that such decisions should not be made by strangers, I advised the parents to find another NICU and another group of neonatologists who would be more receptive to their concerns.

Whatever my own views on the subject may be, we all should be troubled if neonatologists will not honestly discuss their position on forgoing treatment with parents like the Smiths because of vague and unarticulated concerns about the law. Furthermore, the law itself is vague and has been infrequently applied to real cases. If we wait for judges or legislators to decide the fate of severely ill or handicapped newborns, we might as well wait for Godot. In the meantime, many infants, parents, family members, nurses, and others will suffer grievously.

Therapeutic Optimism and the Alteration of the Truth

The parents in this case were not only disqualified by the physicians from participation in decision making about their own son's medical treatment and belatedly confronted with a mysterious policy that forbade any consideration of withdrawing treatment from Cory, but they also were denied the whole truth about his condition. At worst, the physicians involved deceived and manipulated them. At best, they did not disclose to the parents all material information about the situation and benevolently altered the content of what they did disclose.

Even assuming that the first attending neonatologist actually did have an honest disagreement with the radiologist about the interpretation of the head ultrasound performed on Day 2, she still had the obligation of informing the parents of the disagreement. It is a sometimes discomforting fact of life that different but equally competent physicians have different opinions and interpretations of the same phenomenon. The simple fact that two physicians disagree about some aspect of a child's condition cannot alone justify withholding this information from the parents. Say the neonatologist thought Cory might need a serious (and not risk-free) surgical procedure and consulted two conscientious and competent pediatric surgeons, one of whom concluded that surgery was indicated and the other concluded the opposite. The neonatologist would not be ethically justified in failing to inform the parents of the second surgeon's opinion merely because she disagreed with it.

Physicians are often tempted to withhold conflicting medical opinions from the parents for fear it will confuse them or undermine their trust and confidence in the medical profession. Perhaps the disclosure might distress or depress them—a form of harm they could be spared by a more judicious disclosure of information. Perhaps in some cases these might constitute compelling reasons to alter the full truth or at least not disclose everything.

However, I do not believe the failure to disclose all information about the nature and extent of Cory's intraventricular hemorrhage can be justified in this case. First, the attending neonatologist knew that this particular bit of information was especially important to the father, who had, after all, requested that the head ultrasound be done as soon as possible after birth. The father plainly wanted to know this information about his son's condition. Second, as the father was a pediatrician, the parents were in a good position to understand the ultrasound results and put them in context.

It is also possible that the neonatologist intentionally withheld the radiologist's interpretation and consciously (or perhaps unconsciously) altered her own interpretation of the ultrasound scan to avoid having to tell the parents something she strongly suspected might lead them to ask that treatment be discontinued, an option that she might have been no more willing to entertain than was the second attending neonatologist. If that intensive care nursery in fact had a policy of not discontinuing treatment, she knew she might have to contend with knowledgeable parents and "enforce" it if she told the parents all that she knew.

In my experience of clinical practice, it is not uncommon for physicians to alter, stretch, or selectively disclose the truth when talking to parents to present a more optimistic view of the medical situation than the unadulterated facts warrant and to spare the parents the unpleasantness of dealing with the more negative reality. I hesitate to call this lying because it is certainly not a malicious and self-serving lie like that told by Iago about Desdemona. But perhaps my hesitation is misplaced. Someone can modify the truth and do harm for benevolent as well as malevolent reasons. Therapeutic and benevolent optimism has a legitimate place in clinical medicine, but it has a seductive power that can fool the best of physicians into using it at the patient's ultimate expense.

In most cases (and I think this is one of them), a physician should not shield parents from the truth, considerately but accurately presented, about their child's medical condition in order to give them a false sense of hope for the child's prospects and to make them artificially feel better about a bad situation. Furthermore, it is even less ethically justifiable for physicians to modify or distort the truth for their own sake—for example, to be spared the difficulty of contending with the response the truth might generate from the parent. This is so irrespective of the nature of the parents' response—whether it is a sob of heartfelt grief or a demand that further treatment be stopped. Of course, we can throw up our hands like Pontius Pilate, querulously ask "What is truth?" and think that such skepticism justifies expedient manipulation of the facts. This attitude has no place in medical practice, where the facts are, to be sure, imperfectly known but where we must act on the facts as they are.

In the last analysis, there should be little room for lying or distortions of the truth by physicians because anything substantially less than the truth is a deadly worm that can consume the very heart of the healing relationship, or at least damage it very badly. If Cory's parents had found out that they had not received the truth about his intraventricular hemorrhage, they easily could have doubted they had received the truth about other aspects of his condition. Trust in a physician can be replaced quickly with doubt, suspicion, and fear, none of which help sick children get better or help parents cope with the anxiety generated by a child's bad health. Furthermore, if Cory's parents decide to have another child in the future, this venture could be poisoned by the fear that other physicians (obstetricians or pediatricians) will not tell them the truth either. It is not an exaggeration to think that one physician being loose with the truth can make a parent or patient suspicious of the honesty of all other physicians.

Finally, the parents deserved a more honest and forthright response from the second attending neonatologist when they expressed their desire on Day 8 that treatment be discontinued. He knew of the "policy" then, but he remained silent. When he belatedly disclosed the policy (though he lacked the courtesy to talk about something so important to the parents in person), he felt no need to explain or justify it, even though the parents deserved both. This is not to say that such a policy is necessarily illegitimate, but certainly parents who raise the issue of forgoing treatment have the right to know about it. Furthermore, in light of the purported existence of this policy, the assurances of the fellow and the original attending neonatologist that "we'll keep reassessing the situation as things progress" rings false as well. Apparently there was no room at this hospital for reassessment if it included terminating treatment; therefore, the parents did not receive the truth from their very first contact with the neonatologists.

Fortunately, Cory's parents were treated far more considerately by the physicians and other providers at the second hospital. There they were brought into the clinical decision-making process, assisted in reflecting on their desire to discontinue treatment, and given the benefit of honest medical opinion about their son's diagnosis and prognosis. The staff lessened the trauma suffered by the Smiths as a result of their son's sudden premature birth, his serious medical problems, his former physicians' clinical and ethical ineptitude, and the decision they made about his medical care.

Conclusion

I hope that the case of Baby Boy Cory is unusual in its most important particulars, but I know that many of its elements are by no means novel. Many babies suffer from Grade IV intraventricular hemorrhages; many, many more are born prematurely. Many others suffer potentially severe neurological and physical damage from genetic defects, perinatal asphyxia, and other causes. For whatever reason, many parents are neither permitted nor encouraged to assume an active role in decision making about the medical care of their child. In addition, they often are not given the information and support they need to understand what is happening medically to their child nor what is happening psychologically and emotionally to them. What I have called therapeutic optimism is certainly not rare, though how often it lapses into serious manipulation of the truth or outright lying by physicians or nurses I do not know. Fear and confusion about the legal aspects of the care of the critically ill newborn is certainly rampant. More could be said about this, but I would like to conclude on a more personal note.

In the course of talking to Dr. and Mrs. Smith about this case, I mentioned that I was a new, first-time father and immediately felt guilty that I had a full-term, apparently normal infant, though nothing they said or did generated that feeling. In the reproduction lottery, I had been lucky and they had not.

As I look upon my now three-month-old daughter, who shows every sign of doing well and developing normally after being born at term, I am deeply grateful to the obstetricians and nurses who took care of her while she was in the womb and to the pediatricians who facilitated her breathing after she swallowed meconium during the birth process. Yet I hope I never meet a physician who will not tell me the truth about her medical problems (no matter how painful this may be) or who tries to make me think I have no part of making decisions about her medical care and her future. In my less charitable moments, I would dispatch such physicians directly to the devil.

I am grateful and relieved that my daughter did not suffer from any of the medical problems Cory had and that she is with me today. As I have said, I still do not know what I would have felt, thought, or done if she had been in Cory's medical condition. I do not know where my love for her would have led us. But despite my continuing ethical, legal, and personal doubts about Cory's case, I do know that I cannot criticize the manner in which the Smiths chose to act in accordance with their love for him.

Notes

I want to thank Robert Nelson, M.D., of the University of California, San Francisco, and Laurie Dorfman, R.N., of the Bioethics Consultation Group for their assistance in preparing this chapter.

1. Joseph Goldstein, Anna Freud, and Albert J. Solnit, *Beyond the Best Interests of the Child* (New York: Free Press, 1979).

2. Earl E. Shelp, *Born to Die? Deciding the Fate of Critically Ill Newborns* (New York: Free Press, 1986).

3. Howard Brody, "Contested Terrain—in the Best Interests of . . . ," *Hastings Center Report* 18(6) (1988): 37–39.

4. William G. Bartholome, "Contested Terrain—in the Best Interests of . . . ," *Hastings Center Report* 18(6) (1988): 39–40.

5. Robert Weir, *Selective Nontreatment of Handicapped Newborns* (New York: Oxford University Press, 1984), 42. This statistic probably is based on data from the late 1970s and may well be outdated by more recent advances in neonatal medicine.

6. "Perinatology/Neonatology and the Law: Looking beyond Baby Doe," in *1988 Year Book of Perinatal/Neonatal Medicine,* ed. M. Klaus and A. Faranoff (Chicago: Year Book Medical Publishers, 1988), 5–10.

7. L. M. Kopelman, T. G. Irons, and A. E. Kopelman, "Neonatologists Judge the 'Baby Doe' Regulations," *New England Journal of Medicine* 318 (1988): 677–83.

*One way in which this second neonatal case differs from the
first is in which of the involved parties favored continued
aggressive treatment. There is another important difference.
In the first case the attending neonatologist refused to consult
the hospital's ethics committee. In this case, ethics
consultation was an ongoing part of the clinical process.*

Neonatal Ethics: Consultation for Patient, Parents and Professionals

Alan R. Fleischman, M.D.

ON March 3, 1987, Jennifer Brown was born at the Weiler
Hospital of the Albert Einstein College of Medicine. Weiler
Hospital is a voluntary hospital, one of the three tertiary-
level centers in the Division of Neonatology of the Albert Einstein
College of Medicine and Montefiore Medical Center Program. Susan
Brown was thirty-eight years old when she became pregnant for the
third time. Her first two pregnancies had resulted in a spontaneous
abortion and an induced abortion. Susan lived alone in a one-bedroom
apartment. She supported herself reasonably well as a legal secretary
and received excellent health care insurance. The father of the baby,
thirty-four years old, did not live with Susan but had been a close
friend and lover for more than three years. When Susan announced
that she wished to have this baby, he was opposed and asked her to
have an abortion. Susan's decision to continue the pregnancy created a
great deal of stress in their relationship and resulted in his drifting
away, even before the birth of Jennifer.

Alan Fleischman is Director of the Division of Neonatology and Professor of Pediatrics at Albert Einstein College of Medicine and Montefiore Medical Center, Bronx,
New York.

71

Susan arrived at the hospital with her membranes ruptured and was in active labor at two o'clock in the morning. Ultrasound examination revealed a twenty-five- to twenty-six-week old fetus in transverse lie (full-term pregnancy is forty weeks). The left arm of the fetus was extruding from the mother's uterus into her vagina, which necessitated immediate delivery. Delivery was accomplished vaginally by breech extraction. Jennifer was 830 grams (1 pound 13 ounces) at birth. She was severely bruised, had low blood pressure, and was in poor condition. Her Apgar score (the tally of the general condition of an infant; 10 is the highest score, and less than 6 is poor) was 2 at one minute after birth and 4 at five minutes. Because Jennifer's blood pressure and color remained poor, an IV catheter was passed into her umbilical vein in the delivery room, and fluids were administered. On admission to the neonatal intensive care unit at thirty minutes of age, her condition was noted to be critical and her prognosis poor. She was placed on a respirator and achieved a good heart rate and good color.

There was no ethics consultation in the labor room between two o'clock and five o'clock in the morning. There was no perceived need, and no one thought about whether or not this newborn should be aggressively managed. At more than twenty-five weeks gestation, she was considered viable. American perinatology has moved in the past decade to resuscitate virtually all potentially viable infants, looking to contemplative ethical analysis only when there is greater certainty as to outcome after assessment of the patient's potential in the nursery. I certainly would not have recommended an ethics consultation during the period of labor management; however, there were probably some ethical questions in the minds of the caregivers from the beginning. Should an emergency cesarean section, with its increased risks to Susan, have been performed in an attempt to deliver her baby more atraumatically? Should that decision be left to the obstetrical professionals, a team of obstetric and neonatal caregivers, or the woman in labor? These questions were never asked outright, but I am certain they were considered.

Jennifer stabilized during her first day of life on the respirator, although she required a large amount of fluid, a blood transfusion, and protein infusion to maintain blood pressure and urine flow. On the second day of life, her respiratory status deteriorated acutely. High pressures on the respirator were required to force oxygen into Jennifer's immature lungs. The increased pressure caused the fragile lungs to tear and allowed air to escape into the space between the lungs and the chest wall, creating bilateral pneumothoraces. Chest tubes were inserted, and the air was drained; yet her blood pressure and oxygen level did not return to normal. Respirator settings were increased, and heart medications were given to maintain blood pressure and to increase the flow of blood to the vital organs. Her kidneys responded to the decreased blood flow by no longer adequately filtering potentially toxic chemicals. Her blood potassium and creatinine rose to levels that potentially jeopardized her heart function. Ultrasound examination of her head, performed because of the propensity of small prematures to bleed into their brains, revealed a substantial amount of blood inside her brain's ventricles, with abnormal dilatation of these chambers.

Over the next several days severe jaundice developed and required four blood-exchange transfusions to lower her serum bilirubin level. By one week of age it was noted on ultrasound that her brain hemorrhage had extended into the substance of the brain, causing destruction of tissue.

No ethics consultation was requested during this first week of Jennifer's life. Treatment was aggressive. Ms. Brown was informed about Jennifer's condition on a daily basis. She was told that her little girl probably would not survive, and if she did, it was likely she would be severely impaired with cerebral palsy and mental retardation. The attending neonatologist, the neonatal fellow, the pediatric residents, and the neonatal nursing staff all shared the facts of the case with Ms. Brown, looking for clues from her to guide their actions. She continued to have hope and wanted Jennifer to survive even if significant impairment resulted. She urged the treatment team to do everything they could for her daughter.

The neonatal attending, a sensitive and concerned physician, was conflicted. She knew that Jennifer's prognosis for survival was poor and, even more important, that her potential for near normal outcome was virtually nil. It was hard to predict how severely affected Jennifer would be, but more likely than not she would have extensive neuromuscular impairment and severe cognitive dysfunction. In similar cases the neonatologist had offered families the option of withholding further treatment or even withdrawing the respirator so that their child would die, because the treatments were considered virtually futile in terms of ultimate survival. On the other hand, the neonatologist had developed a bond with Susan Brown, a woman unusual in her maturity, her articulateness, and her desire for an infant. The neonatologist wanted to fulfill Susan's desire to take home her baby. Although the information given to Susan was accurate, the uncertainty about Jennifer's outcome was described in more optimistic terms than might have been the case with a mother holding a different view. The neonatologist did not want to take away all hope of survival from this mother who so desperately wanted her baby to live. The situation was ironic: the neonatologist believed it was better if Jennifer did not survive because of her future predicted quality of life, yet the information being conveyed to Susan, the ultimate decision maker, was somewhat slanted in favor of Jennifer's continued aggressive treatment.

During her second and third weeks of life, Jennifer became much less active. It was noted on repeat ultrasound examinations that the fluid-filled chambers inside the brain, the ventricles, were increasing in size, and the substance of the brain was not only being compressed but had areas of severe damage and cell destruction. In addition, she began to have seizures which needed to be controlled with phenobarbital. Nevertheless, to everyone's surprise, Jennifer came off the ventilator on her eighteenth day of life. This was astounding since she had been so critically ill, and it greatly reinforced her mother's belief that she would continue to do better than the medical staff predicted. Jennifer was started on several medications in an attempt to arrest the growing amount of fluid in her brain. At the same time, serial spinal taps were initiated to try to decrease the pressure on her brain and clear the fluid.

At three weeks of age the attending neonatologist had a more formal meeting with Ms. Brown to discuss the serious implications of the increasing fluid in the brain, the already evident brain damage, and the long-term prognosis for Jennifer. At this point Jennifer was breathing comfortably on her own, off the respirator, and decisions about management of the increasing fluid in her brain had to be discussed. Susan continued to insist that she wanted everything done for her baby. She was optimistic that Jennifer would not only survive but do well; regardless, she wanted to take a baby home to love and care for. She stated openly that this might be her last pregnancy and perhaps her last opportunity to have an infant at all. The staff thought that Susan was denying the severity of Jennifer's problems and her likely prognosis in order to cope with the daily stresses of learning about her daughter's course. At the same time, there was some slight possibility that Jennifer would do better than predicted, and Susan continued to focus on that possibility.

Despite careful treatment with medications and repeated spinal taps, the fluid in Jennifer's brain continued to increase. A neurosurgical consultation was requested, and a sampling of fluid directly from the ventricular space in the brain was obtained. The ventricular fluid was thick and brown as a result of the blood that had previously been in the ventricles. After removal of a small quantity of this fluid Jennifer became more alert and responsive. Because the fluid was thick, it would probably not be absorbed by the body on its own, so a treatment plan was developed that included serial ventricular taps to remove fluid and then surgical insertion of an external drainage device to remove the fluid and decrease the compression of the surrounding brain. This plan necessitated transferring Jennifer from the Weiler Hospital to another of the tertiary-level nurseries, North Central Bronx Hospital, where neonatal neurosurgery is performed.

This treatment plan and the questions that were raised by the physicians who would receive Jennifer at the North Central Bronx Hospital initiated the first ethics consultation in this case. The consultation was short and simple. It was carried out on the telephone between the attending neonatologist at the Weiler Hospital and me. Perhaps I should digress for a moment in telling this story to explain who I am and to describe our neonatal ethics consultation program.

I am a neonatologist who has had training in clinical ethics. Over the past ten years I have devoted a substantial amount of time and effort to the field of bioethics and to the teaching of ethical analysis to physicians and nurses. I am responsible for the Infant Bioethics Program in the four hospitals affiliated with the Albert Einstein College of Medicine and the Montefiore Medical Center. I also direct the Division of Neonatology for the Department of Pediatrics. Thus, the attending neonatologists for whom I perform ethics consultations are also part of a division for which I am administratively responsible. To my knowledge, this has not been a significant problem either in terms of ethics consultations or the relationship of division chief to attending physician. This is perhaps because of the openness and feelings of mutual respect among all of the faculty within the division. However, there are some potential conflicts of interest inherent in my dual role as well as some serious questions concerning the autonomous decisions of the clinicians. One might hypothesize that fewer consultations would be requested because of concerns by the attending physicians that their actions might be criticized by their boss. In reality, consultations are requested frequently, and the attendings bring ethical questions to me on virtually a daily basis.

My usual approach is to determine first the medical facts, which my background in clinical neonatology assists me in doing. After doing that in Jennifer's case, I then asked the important question: what is the prognosis as estimated by the attending neonatologist, the neurologist, and the neurosurgeon? All agreed that the likelihood of a good long-term outcome was very slight, but the level of certainty of their predictions varied. The neonatologist and neurologist were very pessimistic. The neurosurgeon, however, recalled one similar patient who did well. He therefore emphasized the quite unlikely but nonetheless possible good outcome for Jennifer. My next question concerned the role of the mother: her level of involvement, the amount and kind of communication that had occurred, her understanding of the future potential of the infant, and her desire for aggressive treatment. I was assured by the attending neonatologist that Ms. Brown wanted everything to be done that might help Jennifer to survive, with the hope that she would do well but with the realistic understanding that this was unlikely. What the attending did not share with me at that point and had not shared with Susan were her personal fears about Jennifer's future. The attending believed that Jennifer would not survive but would die only after having suffered through an unsuccessful series of medical and surgical interventions directed at her progressive brain problem. This was based on the attending's experience with several similar infants and her pessimism about the success of neurosurgical intervention in such small and immature infants. It is likely that the attending did not voice these feelings to me because she knew I would concur, and might push her to share her reservations with Ms. Brown and then reassess whether it was in Jennifer's best interests to proceed with the neurosurgical treatment. Finally, the attending did not share with Susan her belief that if Jennifer did survive she would be at best severely retarded and virtually vegetative. This was, again, based on her experience and on data from the literature but could not be predicted with absolute certainty.

As a consultant I reviewed the facts, the communication with the mother, and the report of the mother's wishes and came to what seemed to be the only possible conclusion: to proceed with aggressive treatment of Jennifer. Through my experience in neonatology and clinical ethics, I have evolved two important and occasionally conflicting principles. The first principle is an infant ought to be provided all forms of care and treatment reasonably thought to be in the infant's best interests. This principle is often utilized in neonatology, but it must be admitted that it is sometimes impossible to determine what is in the best interests of an infant. When there are various options that are in the interests of the child or when it is uncertain what is in the best interests of the child, there must be a method to decide what should be done. This procedural concern is the genesis of the second principle: that the parents bear the moral and decision-making responsibility for their infant and should be the decision makers unless they choose a course of action that is clearly against the infant's best interests. My general approach in consultation, then, has been to empower the parents with decisional authority unless their decisions appear clearly to be against the infant's interests.

This approach bestows a tremendous amount of responsibility on the parents. Some have argued that parents do not have adequate medical knowledge to participate in these best-interests judgments; others have commented that parents might be biased against the interests of their infant because of their own personal pain and suffering or anticipation of future consequences. It has been my experience and observation that virtually all parents are capable of understanding the complexity of neonatal illness and of weighing the treatment options, including the potential for withholding or withdrawing medical intervention. Mothers of all ages, races, and educational and ethnic backgrounds have been able to comprehend and participate in a meaningful way in decisions about their neonates. Of course, it takes a great deal of time, effort, and patience to explain scientifically complex material to parents. It often requires several reiterations over many days, but the vast majority of parents can ultimately understand and integrate the material into their own value systems for decision making.

There are occasional parents who for various reasons are psychologically or socially incapacitated and are unfit surrogates for their children. In such cases, there does not exist a loving parent to weigh options and to choose what is best for the child. My bias in such cases is to recommend in favor of aggressive treatment when what is best for the infant is uncertain, with the belief that we should be in favor of sustaining life unless continued life is burdened by inordinate pain and suffering or is without potential for participation in even the most basic of human interactions.

Susan Brown was clearly a mature, highly involved, concerned, and loving parent. As ethics consultant I learned that Ms. Brown had been informed of all of the treatment options, including stopping, and that she wished the most aggressive management to treat Jennifer's brain problem. She hoped that this would result in both survival and, even though unlikely, normal outcome.

Had Ms. Brown requested no further aggressive treatment for Jennifer, with the likelihood that Jennifer would die, an Infant Bioethics Committee would have been convened to review the ethical appropriateness of the patient's wishes and to ensure that they were consistent with the extant laws and regulations, which will be discussed later. I cannot be certain what the committee would have recommended, but as a member I would have viewed the potential outcome for Jennifer as bleak and the interventions themselves as multiple and painful with little hope for ultimate success. Thus, not being certain what was in Jennifer's best interests, believing that the treatments were virtually futile in terms of her survival, and knowing that the procedures were painful as well, I would have agreed to support Ms. Brown's decision. This was irrelevant because the decision was to continue maximal treatment.

Jennifer was transferred to the North Central Bronx Hospital (NCB) neonatal intensive care unit on March 24 at approximately three weeks of age. She was not on a respirator, but she received oxygen through a nasal tube with constant positive airway pressure. Medical management of the fluid on her brain was continued, and repeat ventricular taps were necessary for decompression. An external drainage system was not inserted because the fluid remained too thick. The neurosurgeons wanted the fluid to be less viscous and cellular prior to inserting an indwelling drainage system; otherwise it would clog up and malfunction.

One week after Jennifer was transferred, her respiratory condition deteriorated. Her lungs, which had been damaged by the early respirator treatment and the need for chest tubes, no longer sustained her ventilation. With her mother's consent, she was reintubated and placed on a respirator on April 1. At this point, Jennifer was constantly uncomfortable. She required frequent suctioning through her breathing tube, which caused coughing; she was stuck for blood tests regularly to assess her breathing status; and a needle had to be placed into her brain every other day to drain off the fluid. She could no longer be held without concern for dislodging the breathing tube, so she was held by her mother and the nurses less frequently. She appeared to be constantly irritable, and medication was used to relieve some of the discomfort.

During that week at NCB Susan visited frequently and came to know the new caregiving team. The original attending neonatologist continued to be involved in Jennifer's care, not as the primary attending but as a concerned and involved consultant to both the treatment team and Ms. Brown. The new attending neonatologist agreed with the aggressive plan of management and, in fact, believed that this was in the best interests of the infant because of the slight possibility that she could survive and do well. The nursing professionals and the resident pediatricians in the neonatal unit were quite concerned that Jennifer would neither survive nor do well based on their experience with many similar children. After the child was reintubated, they sought another ethics consultation.

The second ethics consultation took place as part of a program called Neonatal Ethics Rounds, which occurs every other week in the neonatal unit at NCB. These rounds include all of the neonatal caregivers, a philosopher, an attorney from the Law and Ethics Program at Montefiore Medical Center, and myself. We again reviewed the facts of the case and the involvement of Ms. Brown in treatment decisions. I personally was becoming far more pessimistic about Jennifer's ability to survive. I was concerned that at this point we were causing undue pain and suffering to both Jennifer and her mother, with essentially no potential for reasonable outcome. I was concerned that the transfer from one hospital to another had resulted in a change in the amount of information that Ms. Brown was receiving. I wanted to be certain that Ms. Brown understood that the recent deterioration and the need to place Jennifer back on the respirator were important in terms of Jennifer's long-term prognosis.

The ethics rounds focused on the important question of how far the neonatal team should go in providing resuscitative measures to Jennifer if her heart slowed or stopped, secondary to the increased pressure on her brain. The residents and nurses caring for Jennifer on a moment-to-moment basis wanted to know if a "do not resuscitate" (DNR) order was appropriate. This question was perhaps based more on the pragmatic need to know what to do in the event of cardiac arrest than on a strongly held belief that resuscitation was wrong. The nursing staff, to a greater extent than the residents, were opposed to resuscitation in the event of sudden cardiac decompensation because of their belief that Jennifer would not ultimately survive regardless of the interventions currently being planned. It was agreed at the neonatal ethics rounds to raise the question of resuscitation with Ms. Brown and to recommend to her that a DNR order be written. This order would not change any of the aggressive treatments being given to Jennifer but would give direction to the caregivers in the event of her heart's completely stopping. The caregivers sought the DNR order because they believed it was in Jennifer's best interests to have all treatment stopped but that Ms. Brown would never agree. They also believed that if the heart slowed or stopped it would be a sign of an even more serious brain malfunction, that further treatment would be futile, and that Jennifer would die regardless of what was done. Therefore, they believed the DNR order was appropriate and that Ms. Brown might be convinced that if Jennifer's heart stopped she should not be resuscitated.

Ms. Brown agreed to a DNR order but still hoped that Jennifer would benefit from aggressive medical and surgical intervention. She agreed that if Jennifer's heart stopped while on the respirator, it would be a sign that Jennifer really could not ultimately survive. Subsequent to the order not to resuscitate, Jennifer had many episodes of slowing of her heart, but it did not completely stop. Each of these episodes was responded to immediately by the doctors and nurses in the neonatal unit with various interventions to restore cardiac rate. Clearly the DNR order was not taken as a license to ignore Jennifer, nor was it taken as an order not to intervene to prevent cardiac arrest. It is interesting that the professionals acted to prevent cardiac arrest even though they believed that survival was not in Jennifer's interests. This was done not out of fear of criticism or legal repercussions but out of a genuine respect for parental discretion in such situations.

Over the next two weeks Jennifer continued on the ventilator with intermittent ventricular taps for decompression of the fluid. She did not tolerate oral feeding and was nourished intravenously through a central catheter. Her weight increased so that by six weeks of age she weighed more than one kilogram (2 pounds, 3 ounces). Her general clinical condition did not improve. She became less responsive and lacked spontaneous activity. The caregivers and Ms. Brown became even less optimistic about Jennifer's long-term prognosis, and a general level of depression ensued. Chart notes and daily work rounds focused on the multiple problems that required meticulous management for Jennifer to survive.

A third ethics consult occurred at approximately seven weeks of life, when a blood culture revealed a generalized systemic infection, and fluid from the ventricular tap showed a change in white blood cell count consistent with infection. Even the most optimistic of the caregivers were devastated by these new findings. Jennifer's chance for survival was virtually nil. She began to have frequent seizures, which previously had been well controlled on phenobarbital. These new convulsions required additional medication. Jennifer became generally moribund and completely unresponsive. All of the caregivers were now in agreement that continued medical intervention was of no benefit to her. Even if the infections could be brought under control, her future survival was doubtful and her brain had been further severely and irreversibly damaged. The purpose of the third consultation was to determine whether the Infant Bioethics Committee agreed that stopping all treatment was appropriate.

I listened to the anger and frustration of the caregivers in describing their guilt in having failed to maintain this infant and their feelings of failure in being unable to give Ms. Brown the child she desired. They wanted the committee to tell them it was okay to stop the ventilator, and they wanted to be able to say to the mother that the Committee had prescribed withdrawal of treatment. I reminded them that the Infant Bioethics Committee was created not to make these decisions but to review them after physicians and parents had decided what they believed to be in the interests of the infant. Alternatively, if there was a conflict between the physicians and parents, the committee would review the issue. Our Infant Bioethics Committee, which by this time had been in existence for over three years, does review ongoing cases; in fact, there is mandatory review of those cases in which it is proposed to withdraw or withhold life-sustaining treatment for a patient who is not otherwise imminently dying.[1] Thus, Jennifer's case would fall within the responsibility of the Infant Bioethics Committee to review. The physicians caring for Jennifer insisted that the mother wanted continued aggressive management, even though they believed it was no longer in Jennifer's interest. This created a conflict between caregivers and mother about what indeed was in the best interests of the child. Because of this conflict situation, a meeting of the Infant Bioethics Committee was called for the following day.

In convening the committee, an interdisciplinary team of physicians, ethicists, lawyers, nurses, social workers, administrators, and lay participants, which I chair, I had several goals. First and foremost was to air Jennifer's case in an objective and thoughtful manner. Second, and perhaps almost as important, I hoped to validate the young professionals' view that they were not obligated to inflict pain and suffering on a child merely because the mother wished such treatment, if there was no potential benefit. The analytic task for the committee would be to determine whether Susan ought to be respected in clinging to some hope, even if slim, that Jennifer might survive, or whether her wishes should be given lower priority because of her denial of the changes in Jennifer's prognosis based on the newly available information.

The committee met at noon and learned about Jennifer's complicated history. The caregivers had requested that Ms. Brown not be invited to the meeting so that they might sort out their own feelings and obligations concerning Jennifer with the committee's help. Several members were especially concerned about the great suffering Jennifer had already endured and the extremely slight chance of any benefit from continued intervention. The committee unanimously agreed that the caregivers should recommend to Ms. Brown that she strongly consider withdrawing the ventilator from Jennifer and allowing her to die. Ms. Brown could choose to be present or not as she wished. The committee also stated that if Ms. Brown did not wish the ventilator withdrawn, the caregivers were obligated to continue all treatments, based on the slim chance that Jennifer might yet survive, because if she survived her outcome would be optimized by continued aggressive management.

As director of neonatology, I had developed in each of our nurseries an area where parents might mourn and grieve at the end of their child's life. Extracted from all of the technology, infants can be held by their parents and, perhaps for the first time, truly comforted. This approach to the end of neonatal life had been observed by several members of the Infant Bioethics Committee and was felt to be a reasonable and appropriate end for Jennifer. It was also thought to be therapeutic for Susan to allow her to be a comforting mother and spend some time with her daughter in a quiet and close final interaction.

At the end of the Infant Bioethics Committee meeting caregivers felt energized in their resolve to discuss these difficult issues with Ms. Brown. Susan knew that the committee had convened and, in fact, was waiting in the nursery for their return from the meeting. The doctors and nurses shared with Susan their belief that continued treatment was hopeless. They strongly recommended that Susan agree to stop the ventilator and allow Jennifer to die. Ms. Brown's response was to request some time to think about it. Her attachment to Jennifer precluded her being able to request or even agree to the withdrawal of the ventilator. She saw this as agreeing to kill Jennifer. All along she had had no problem with letting Jennifer die if her heart stopped or if treatment was not successful. At this point the physicians were asking her not only to let Jennifer die but to hasten that death by withdrawal of treatment. Susan went home to think; she had dinner and returned to the hospital in the evening.

Very depressed, Susan sat at Jennifer's bedside. She could not acquiesce to the cessation of the ventilator. Jennifer began to have severe slowing of her heart. The nurses and doctors at the bedside, with Susan present, did not respond by increasing the ventilator setting or giving medications, as they had in the past. Susan was aware that they were letting Jennifer die and said nothing. She could not acquiesce, but she did not object. As Jennifer's color changed, Susan sat weeping and being comforted by the nurse. Finally, Jennifer's heart stopped. No resuscitative efforts were made, and a few minutes later the nurses took Jennifer off all of the monitoring equipment, wrapped her in a baby blanket, and let Susan hold her unencumbered for the first time.

This case, more than many others in which I have been involved, created serious questions for me as ethics consultant, neonatologist, and medical educator. Based on my personal experience and knowledge of the literature, I would have predicted when Jennifer was two days old that because of her devastating level of illness she would either not survive or would survive with severe neurological damage. These data and biases would not have resulted in my recommendation of cessation of treatment but would have made my discussions with Jennifer's family very pessimistic and couched in negative terms. Is this fair to future unborn neonates? What level of certainty about outcome is required before a pessimistic view is presented? Is it the obligation of the clinician to share information on a statistical probability basis, giving no personal interpretations of these value-laden data?

Some have argued that the recent federal interest in neonatal treatment and the federal regulations that were put into effect in 1985[2] preclude any considerations about withholding or withdrawing medical interventions from infants unless they are imminently dying. My reading of the Child Abuse Amendment and of the regulations that place responsibility for supervision of decision making with each state's Child Protection Services Agency is that it is still incumbent on clinicians and parents to make difficult ethical judgments for critically ill neonates. The Child Abuse Amendment states that a treating physician's reasonable medical judgment must be utilized in determining what is appropriate nutrition, hydration, and medication for each infant. It should be assumed that such appropriate treatments are mandatory except in three specific instances: when the infant is irreversibly comatose, when the provision of such treatment would merely prolong the dying process, and when the provision of such treatment would be virtually futile in terms of the survival of the infant and the treatment itself under such circumstances would be inhumane. A substantial proportion of the treatments of critically ill infants in neonatal units may be inhumane and virtually futile in terms of the infant's survival. Many of the treatments that Jennifer received subsequent to the decision to aggressively treat her severe and progressive brain problem were virtually futile in terms of her survival, and because of the pain and suffering they inflicted on her they could be considered inhumane.

How should physicians and nurses make reasonable medical judgments concerning which treatments should be recommended, which are virtually futile, and which prolong the inevitable dying of an infant? I have no easy answer for this most difficult of questions. But if treatments are virtually futile in terms of survival, I utilize parental discretion as a determinant of which treatments ought to be pursued. I can think of no better way to make these incredibly complex and value-laden choices than to respect the choice of the mother from whose body the infant has recently been born. I believe in the principle that those who bear the burden of a decision ought to have a significant role in making it. However, I believe that parents should be more than just involved in such critical decisions; their choices should be respected as determinative whenever treatments are virtually futile and offer little potential benefit for the child.

When should a parent's judgment concerning her infant be questioned? The easy answer is, when the choice is not in the infant's best interest. The hard part is defining when that occurs. It is simple for those of us caring for an infant with Down's syndrome and a blockage in the intestines to argue that parents who would choose death rather than a simple surgical intervention are not acting in their infant's interests, and their refusal of treatment ought to be overridden. It is more difficult, when caring for a critically ill and dying infant for whom you believe treatment is only causing pain and suffering with no compensating benefit, to respect a parent's choice to continue treatment. Medical caregivers should not merely be technologists, carrying out the wishes of their patients or their patients' families. Our society ought not wish such automatons at the bedside nor should medical and nursing professionals be encouraged to leave their consciences at home and perform their skills unquestioningly.

It is my goal as an ethics consultant to point out these inherent

tensions between the roles and responsibilities of the medical professionals and the roles and responsibilities of the parents. These tensions
ought to benefit the infant by creating an environment of collaborative
decision making among the many people who are concerned about the
well-being of this very vulnerable and fragile patient. Simple answers—
like treating all infants at all times or respecting parental decisions
without question—will not result in the best outcomes for the most
infants. Complex answers arrived at in a thoughtful manner while
respecting parental discretion, such as in the case of Jennifer Brown,
are by far preferable to quick decisions concerning withholding or
withdrawing treatments or never considering these options.

As a neonatologist and as an ethics consultant I feel it is my responsibility to share with other professionals and with parents the personal
pain I have experienced as a result of aiding in the survival of infants
for whom the outcomes have been abysmal. Some have argued that, in
America, allowing the death of an infant who otherwise would have
survived and been normal is a far greater evil than forcing an infant to
live who becomes a severely disabled and handicapped infant with
little potential for cognitive development. For me, one is not worse
than the other; both are terrible outcomes. Physicians, nurses, and
therapists in the neonatal intensive care unit must not feel an obligation to send home only infants who would have the potential to develop
into a so-called normal child. It is not our job to guarantee that all
graduates of our neonatal units are healthy and happy infants. However, we should neither impose our own values on our patients and
their parents nor refrain from sharing our knowledge, experience, and
feelings with them.

The goal of an ethics consultant is to ensure that all of the medical,
psychological, and value-laden facts are before those who are responsible for the care and the decision making in the neonatal unit. With the
neonate as the center of the focus, the best-interests standard ought to
be applied. When what is in the best interests of the infant cannot
clearly be determined, parents should be given great discretion. The
ethics consultant and/or the Infant Bioethics Committee can assure
that the appropriate facts have been obtained and the appropriate
process has occurred.

I believe this occurred in Jennifer Brown's case. Whether or not it
would have been better for Jennifer to have lived a little longer or died a
little sooner, the caregivers and her mother made thoughtful and considered judgments that they felt were in Jennifer's best interests. The

small role that the ethics consultations played was to help the clinicians reflect on the reasons for their choices and on the boundaries of parental decision making in Jennifer's care. I hope I was also able to give some ethical comfort to the grieving staff and through them to Jennifer's mother.

Notes

1. Alan R. Fleischman, "Bioethical Review Committee in Perinatology," *Clinics in Perinatology* 14 (1987): 379–93.
2. U.S. Department of Health and Human Services, "Child Abuse and Neglect Prevention and Treatment Program," *Federal Register* 50 (1985): 14878–901.

We return to a case involving an adult patient, a patient who suffered from an unusual, little-known, and frightening malady. The author, because of circumstance, acted as both treating physician and ethics consultant.

Ethical Considerations in the Locked-in Syndrome

James L. Bernat, M.D.

M. Noirtier, immovable as a corpse, looked at the new-comers with a quick and intelligent expression, perceiving at once by their ceremonious courtesy, that they were come on business of an unexpected and official character. Sight and hearing were the only senses remaining, and they appeared left, like two solitary sparks, to animate the miserable body which seemed fit for nothing but the grave; it was only, however, by means of one of these senses that he could reveal the thoughts and feelings which still worked in his mind, and the look by which he gave expression to this inner life resembled one of those distant lights which are sometimes seen in perspective by the benighted traveller while crossing some cheerless desert, apprising him that there is still another human being who is awake in that silence and darkness . . . in short his whole appearance produced on the mind the impression of a corpse with living eyes.[1]

I N *The Count of Monte-Cristo* (1845), Alexandre Dumas gave this description of M. Noirtier de Villefort, probably the earliest account of the tragic disorder now known as the locked-in syndrome. Like the usual locked-in case, M. Noirtier was totally paralyzed and mute but fully alert mentally and able to communicate by opening and clos-

James Bernat is Professor of Clinical Medicine (Neurology) at Dartmouth Medical School, Hanover, New Hampshire, and Chief of the Neurology Section, Veterans Administration Medical Center, White River Junction, Vermont.

ing his eyes. The term "locked-in" was applied to this syndrome in 1966 by Plum and Posner, who described a typical case and emphasized the psychological implications of awake but profoundly paralyzed and mute patients.[2] Several hundred locked-in cases have been reported subsequently.

The pathologic lesion producing the locked-in syndrome is usually a stroke involving the brain stem, a part of the central nervous system between the spinal cord and the midbrain. Specifically, it is an infarction (the blockage of a blood vessel) or hemorrhage (the bursting of a blood vessel) in the pons.[3] Many large nerve pathways coursing through the pons are interrupted, producing complete paralysis of voluntary movements of the face, larynx, trunk, and limbs. Horizontal eye movements are absent because of the destruction of the pontine gaze centers. Vertical eye movements are preserved because their pathways are all outside the pons and are unaffected by the lesion. Voluntary eyelid opening and closing is usually preserved. Locked-in patients remain awake, with full awareness, sentience, and cognition (intellectual abilities), because the centers for consciousness and cognition are unaffected. Electroencephalograms of locked-in patients are normal, reflecting their preserved cognition.[4] Similar syndromes of mental alertness with profound paralysis may be seen occasionally in patients with other neurological diseases.

The prognosis in locked-in syndrome from pontine infarction is generally poor, although several cases with good recovery have been reported.[5] If recovery is going to occur, the first evidence of improvement is usually seen during the first few months. As a result, most physicians prefer to treat locked-in patients aggressively, at least initially. Most patients with large pontine strokes remain locked-in or progress to coma and death. Patients may remain locked-in for over a decade.

Communication for these patients is possible only with the use of vertical eye and eyelid movements. Several patients reportedly have been taught to communicate by Morse code, using vertical eye movements.[6] At least one locked-in patient has "dictated" a book by this method. Dumas described M. Nortier looking down and closing his eyes to signify disapproval of a question posed to him and opening his eyes and looking up to signify approval. In this manner, he was able to actively control and even manipulate his family.

A host of important ethical issues is raised in the diagnosis and management of locked-in patients. I recently served as neurological and ethics consultant to a patient who progressed from the locked-in syndrome to coma and death. He posed several challenging ethical problems.

Case Report

Mr. Webb was sixty-five years old when he was admitted for treatment of severe breathing difficulty. He had been a heavy cigarette smoker for many years and suffered from advanced chronic obstructive pulmonary disease with heart failure. His past medical history also included obesity, hypertension, and moderate alcohol use. He was a divorced dairy farmer, had three grown children, and lived alone. Inpatient treatment with respiratory therapy, oxygen, steroids, and intravenous bronchodilators produced a marked improvement in his shortness of breath by the third hospital day.

While undergoing respiratory therapy on the fourth hospital day, he suddenly became rigid and unresponsive. My neurological examination thereafter disclosed a sweating, obese, red-faced man who was clearly awake and alert but profoundly paralyzed and mute. He was breathing regularly at a slightly increased rate. He lay motionless except for breathing. His pupils were small and constricted when light was shone in his eyes. He was unable to move his face, limbs, or trunk voluntarily. Eye movements in the horizontal plane were absent, both voluntarily and reflexively; he could voluntarily move his eyes only in the vertical plane. Corneal reflexes (involuntary blinking when the surface of the eye is touched) were absent. He could neither speak nor make any sounds, but his hearing was intact. He could not swallow, and all of his limbs were paralyzed. Sensation to painful stimuli was apparently preserved in all four limbs and in his trunk.

The clinical diagnosis was locked-in syndrome from a pontine infarction. A tomography (CT) brain scan confirmed the diagnosis. Mr. Webb remained alert and attentive and was clearly aware of himself and his predicament. Although paralyzed and mute, he was able to communicate by making vertical eye movement responses to "yes–no" questions. When we informed him of our uncertainty about his prognosis, he indicated that he wished to be treated aggressively. Much effort was spent educating the medical and nursing staff about techniques for communicating with him as he used his vertical eye and eyelid movements to signify yes and no. Plans were made to insert a gastrostomy tube (a tube inserted surgically directly into the stomach for liquid feeding) and to arrange for long-term placement. His neurological examination remained unchanged for two days.

On the sixth hospital day, he suddenly stopped breathing and had a convulsive seizure. He was quickly resuscitated and placed on a mechanical ventilator. Neurological examination then revealed a deeply comatose man who did not breathe spontaneously. He lay motionless with his eyes closed and made no response whatsoever to verbal stimuli. His pupils were pinpoint in diameter and reacted to light, but there were no voluntary or reflex horizontal *or* vertical movements of the eyes when eye movements were stimulated through appropriate testing. A second CT brain scan was unchanged from two days earlier.

I thought his pontine infarction had extended and was now producing deep coma in addition to the other signs of profound brain stem dysfunction. Our plan was to treat aggressively for seventy-two hours to assess his stability and to determine whether this new development was reversible. His daughter, the next of kin, was contacted. She met with the treating physicians, another ethics consultant, and me. She consulted her two siblings and the patient's brother, his only sibling. They decided immediately to declare him do-not-resuscitate: if his heart stopped, no attempt would be made to restart it. We decided that he should remain intubated and ventilated until I could be more certain that he had a hopeless prognosis.

My repeat neurological examination four days after the onset of coma showed no improvement. He remained deeply comatose, and his brain stem functioning appeared even worse than four days earlier. By this time I felt that I could predict with reasonable certainty that he would not recover consciousness, regardless of the aggressiveness or duration of our treatment.

The daughters and son discussed Mr. Webb's poor prognosis in the context of their understanding of their father's previously stated wishes. All three children agreed that their father would want to have his treatment terminated in his present situation, given the poor prognosis. To illustrate their father's value system, they told a story. Several months earlier, a close friend died; she had been unconscious and on a ventilator for two weeks before her death. Mr. Webb told his eldest daughter that he did not want this type of lingering dying to happen to him. Rather, if there were no hope for his recovery, he wanted his death to be "quick and easy." The family and I discussed the discontinuation of his current therapies in light of his previously expressed wishes. All agreed to stop his ventilator, his medications, and his supplemental oxygen. Withdrawal of hydration and nutrition was not discussed. I believed that because of his need for the ventilator he would die within a short time of its withdrawal. There was unanimous agreement with this plan by his treating physicians, the other ethics consultant, the nurses, the patient's three children, his brother, and me.

The afternoon of the tenth hospital day, he was taken off the ventilator, and all medications and oxygen were withdrawn. Hydration and nutrition were maintained. Mr. Webb died quietly from respiratory failure four hours later. Permission was not granted for an autopsy.

Comment

Mr. Webb's unfortunate case raises several interesting issues: (1) the ethical problems posed by the locked-in patient, (2) how decision making regarding the aggressiveness of treatment of patients with brain damage depends largely upon the prognosis; (3) the role of the ethics consultant in the management of the locked-in patient; (4) how decision making can be performed successfully for permanently incompetent patients, and (5) what case law exists regarding decision making for locked-in patients.

Ethical Problems of the Locked-in Patient

The particular ethical problems arising in patients with locked-in syndrome result from the unique features of this disorder. Such patients are awake, fully conscious, and mentally intact. Yet they are profoundly paralyzed and unable to vocalize; they can successfully communicate only with the assistance, patience, and dedication of other people. It is no exaggeration to describe the plight of the locked-in patient, as Dumas did, as an alert mind imprisoned in a useless body.

To place their condition into a more familiar context, one is tempted to compare locked-in patients to those rendered quadriplegic from a cervical spinal cord injury. But the plight of the locked-in patient is far worse. First, communication is immensely more difficult for the locked-in patient. Second, pain sensation remains intact, and as a result, the locked-in patient is capable of profound suffering. For example, the locked-in patient may be lying in an uncomfortable position yet be unable to move or to communicate his discomfort. Third, it is much more difficult for locked-in patients to manipulate their environment effectively.

The locked-in patient may be mistakenly regarded as unconscious by

the unwary examiner. We all evidence our consciousness and awareness through our responses to verbal and other external stimuli, so it is
difficult for the mute, profoundly paralyzed, brain-damaged patient to
convince the examiner that he is awake and attentive. I have examined
several locked-in patients who previously had been regarded as comatose by their treating physicians. Because of the resemblance to coma in
these cases, the medical and nursing staff had made no attempt to
communicate with the patients or to consider them conscious and in
pain or discomfort. Conversations had been clearly heard that staff had
thought were uttered over an unconscious patient. The error of treating
an awake and cognitive person as unconscious compounds the already
enormous suffering experienced by locked-in patients.

The macabre condition of the awake but paralyzed patient was cap-
tured in an episode of Rod Serling's *Twilight Zone*, originally aired
around 1960. A man was critically injured in an automobile accident.
He was wide awake, but because of his profound paralysis and mute-
ness he was mistakenly thought to be hopelessly comatose by his
treating physician. His only remaining voluntary motor response to
demonstrate his conscious state was his ability to wiggle his left little
finger. Unhappily, his left hand was out of sight under a sheet. The
victim's overwhelming frustration, fear, and agony were clearly por-
trayed as he heard his physician state that he was comatose and that his
case was hopeless. At about the time the physician was considering
declaring him dead, the patient shed a tear, alerting the physician to the
life and consciousness present in the patient. Because of similar frus-
trations, many locked-in patients also cry tears. In a similar vein, Edgar
Allen Poe often employed the theme of the agony of the awake, conscious person who is mistakenly declared dead and buried.

In Mr. Webb's case, his physicians and nurses alertly recognized his
locked-in state and treated him as awake from the beginning. He was
gently told that he had suffered a stroke rendering him paralyzed and
mute, but that we all knew he was awake and mentally intact. Considerable efforts were made to communicate with him using his eye open-
ings and vertical movements as signals for yes and no. Attempts were
made to assess and enhance his degree of comfort.

As is true in the majority of locked-in patients, Mr. Webb remained
competent throughout the time he was locked in. Brain centers for
awareness, alertness, and cognition are not usually damaged in the
locked-in syndrome, so there is no diminution of intelligence or competence as a result of the disorder. Therefore, the same standards govern-

ing decision making by any competent patient also applied to Mr. Webb. Simply stated, we physicians were ethically bound to follow Mr. Webb's rational health care decisions.[7]

Of course, Mr. Webb's ability to communicate was severely impaired. Explaining his disease and gaining assurance that he had understood us was difficult and time-consuming. We believed that by his yes and no signals he could communicate his understanding of his condition and his decisions regarding the aggressiveness of our treatment. But it was much more difficult for us to be certain that he understood than it would have been with a patient who could respond by speech and gesture. Often, we had to repeat our questions to him several times or phrase them in different ways to feel confident that he understood them and was able to provide consistent answers. Even then, we often could not be certain. For this reason, our ability to judge the quality of the consent process is necessarily limited in the locked-in patient.

The Role of the Ethics Consultant for the Locked-in Patient

The role of the ethics consultant in Mr. Webb's case was to assure that his physicians treated him the same as any other competent patient: his rational choices regarding his own health care would be followed. He was educated about his condition, particularly about his prognosis. He was told that most people with pontine strokes producing the locked-in syndrome do not recover, but some people do recover. He was given the option of cardiopulmonary resuscitation. He was instructed that he would require a feeding gastrostomy tube because of his inability to swallow. His physicians were forthright but encouraging and supportive. He was assured that his physicians would perform whatever treatment was necessary to keep him comfortable and healthy pending the hoped-for recovery. As ethics consultant, I made it clear to his other physicians that the treatment choices were squarely his own to make, given the necessary information and support. After considering this information and advice, Mr. Webb chose full support, including candidacy for cardiopulmonary resuscitation, and these wishes were followed.

Mr. Webb remained conscious for only two days before his brain stem stroke was extended and he became deeply comatose. However, other locked-in patients have remained in a stable paralyzed state for many months to years. Given the total dependency and hopelessness of such patients, it is common for them to become depressed. If a previously courageous locked-in patient changes his mind and wishes to die, he should receive psychiatric evaluation and treatment for pre-sumed depression. In the absence of evidence for the diagnosis of depression, if the patient expresses a consistent wish to die and refuses medical treatment to that end, his refusal of treatment is valid and should be respected.

I believe that the wish to die as the only means to escape a perma-nently locked-in existence counts as a rational decision. If one's life can never be more than permanent dependency, suffering, and pain, with-out the countervailing benefits of hope for improvement and physical independence, one has an adequate reason to refuse life-sustaining treatment, including hydration and nutrition. The well-publicized case of Elizabeth Bouvia contains many similarities to the patient with the locked-in syndrome who refuses treatment, although her neurological deficits are not as profound.

In my role as ethics consultant, I helped outline the decision-making process regarding the appropriate level of care for Mr. Webb when he became comatose and it was clear that he would not recover con-sciousness. I discovered that he had left no advance directives pertain-ing to his current predicament but had discussed an analogous situa-tion with his daughter and told her how he would want to be treated in such a state. I explained to the family that the decision of whether to continue or terminate treatment should be made on the basis of trying to find and follow the decision that Mr. Webb would have made if, magically, he were temporarily competent to do so. It was on the basis of this "substituted judgment" that the children were to decide for their father. Put into these terms, it was easier for them to accept the decision for nontreatment because doing so was following Mr. Webb's previ-ously stated wishes.

The Role of Prognosis in Decision Making

In the two stages of Mr. Webb's neurological illness he received vastly different levels of aggressiveness of treatment. Initially, he received full therapeutic support, including candidacy for cardiopulmonary resus-citation. This treatment plan was appropriate because Mr. Webb had made a valid consent for it, based largely, I believe, on the hope that he would be one of the minority of locked-in patients who would recover. But this plan was not irrevocable. If, after several weeks or months, he did not begin to show evidence for recovery, he had the option of changing the degree of aggressiveness of treatment. We would have been obligated to follow the new, lessened treatment plan as a rational decision made by a competent patient.

As it happened, his stroke progressed to include the ascending reticular formation, the center for wakefulness in the brain stem. When, because of his continued neurologic deterioration, it became clear that he was permanently comatose, his family decided that he would not want to continue living in this manner. At that point, treatments that had been ordered were withdrawn. The same treatments that earlier had been appropriate because of their contribution to his hoped-for personal health goals now were no longer appropriate because the treatments could not possibly attain those goals.

Mr. Webb's example shows how prognosis can be a critical factor in a patient's choice of desired levels of treatment. This relationship between prognosis and treatment choice is almost always present for patients with disorders of the central nervous system and is usually present for patients with disorders of other bodily systems. The prognosis for recovery of consciousness is a watershed in decision making for the patient with a neurological disorder. Once the prognosis is confidently made that there is little or no probability of regaining consciousness, most persons say they would want to be allowed to die. Consciousness is probably the critical factor in personhood.[8] If it is irreversibly lost, medical therapeutics seem worthless. Most people assign little value to the maintenance of a permanently noncognitive, vegetative existence.

Decision Making for Permanently Incompetent Patients

When patients become permanently incompetent, their health care decisions must be made by others serving as proxy decision makers. The proxies should attempt to use the standard of substituted judgment, which requires the proxy to make the same decision that the patient would have made in the given situation if he or she were still competent. Successfully fulfilling the standard of substituted judgment requires a clear knowledge of the patient's values and choices. Mr. Webb's daughters were able to successfully fulfill this standard because they had recently discussed his personal feelings about a mutual friend in a similar situation. The substituted judgment standard permits the ethical and legal principle of self-determination to be exercised even after the person has become permanently incompetent.

The presence of advance directives assists the proxy in fulfilling the goal of substituted judgment. If written advance directives had been executed by Mr. Webb, their existence would have provided additional information concerning his specific wishes for treatment in various situations. Most currently written advance directives, however, contain language that is so vague that proxies are required to interpret them by applying their knowledge of the patient's values to the specific situation. We should have discussed with Mr. Webb what level of treatment he would desire were he to become incompetent. Because he was locked in for only two days, most of the time was spent communicating with him about his immediate treatment.

When no information exists to permit a decision by substituted judgment, the "best interest" standard should be used. Here, proxies must use their own system of values to decide what, in their opinion, is in the best interest of the patient. The best-interest standard is not as ethically powerful as the substituted-judgment standard because it requires the application of another person's value system which may or may not be the same as that of the patient. Fortunately, it was not necessary for the family to apply the best-interest standard for Mr. Webb.

The Treating Physician as Ethics Consultant

In this case I functioned both as a treating physician and as one of the two ethics consultants. This dual role is unusual in larger hospitals but does occur in small hospitals such as ours. In our hospital I am one of the two primary ethics consultants and the only full-time neurologist.

It is difficult for me to see that I had any serious conflicts in filling both roles. I believe I was able to execute both responsibilities adequately. By having experience in both neurological and ethical matters, I was in a unique position to provide care to a patient in the locked-in syndrome.

To pursue further the question of dual-consultant conflicts of interest, consider the situation in which an internist with specialty training in gastroenterology is treating a hospitalized patient for pneumonia. If the patient subsequently develops acute gastrointestinal bleeding, the internist can function also as the patient's gastroenterologist and treat the bleeding. I see no necessity for the internist to consult another gastroenterologist because of a conflict of interests.

Yet ethics consultations are different from medical consultations. One potential area of conflict surrounds the maintenance of objectivity in the mind of the treating physician when he or she also serves as ethics consultant. Emotional involvement may render the physician less objective than is optimal for an ethics consultant. Another potential area of conflict is the requirement of the ethics consultant to be a dispassionate advocate for the patient. Treating physicians who develop strong opinions about patient management based on certain past experiences or fears may no longer be capable of functioning in a disinterested capacity, even though they may believe they are doing so.

In small hospitals such as ours, this dual role may be inevitable at times. A reasonable safeguard to help guarantee objectivity is to seek the advice of another ethics consultant in cases in which the primary ethics consultant has a dual role. In Mr. Webb's case, the two ethics consultants were in agreement. In hospitals in which there is only one ethics consultant available, review with another physician is a reasonable practice.

Judicial Precedents for Decision Making in Locked-in Patients

There are two high court precedents granting locked-in patients the authority to refuse life-sustaining treatments. In the Rodas case, a thirty-four-year-old man in a locked-in syndrome from brain stem stroke requested termination of all life-sustaining treatments, including hydration and nutrition. This right was upheld by the Colorado District Court, which found the decision "rational and reasonable" and ruled that the patient was mentally capable of refusing treatment.[9] In the Putzer case, the Superior Court of New Jersey permitted a sixty-five-year-old man, in a locked-in syndrome from a brain stem infarction, to die by refusing all therapies, including hydration and nutrition.[10] Both courts held that competent patients had the right to refuse therapies even if that refusal produced their deaths, that it counted as a rational choice to want to die if permanently in the locked-in syndrome, and that such decisions did not constitute suicide. Both courts used ethical analyses in their arguments, in particular the overriding importance of the rights of competent patients to consent to or refuse proposed treatments.

Afterword

I feel that our management of Mr. Webb was satisfactory by both ethical and neurological standards. I regret that during his two days in the locked-in syndrome we did not discuss with him his feelings about living or dying were he subsequently to become irreversibly comatose. We should have tried to discover these wishes because it would have made us more confident in the ethical soundness of our withdrawal of care and would have relieved his children of making what was for them a difficult decision.

Perhaps we chose not to discuss the possibility of a bad outcome with him because of our own psychological discomfort about initiating such a discussion. However, I think the main reason we did not discuss with him the possibility of progression to coma was our desire not to discourage him after he had made such a courageous decision to press onward with aggressive treatment.

By his spontaneous progression to coma and our subsequent termination of his treatment, Mr. Webb spared us from a later, more difficult problem. What if, after being locked in for several months without improvement, Mr. Webb decided to refuse all further treatment, including hydration and nutrition, and wanted to be permitted to die? I would have felt a strong moral obligation to carry out this wish because of my duty to respect the rational wishes of a competent patient. There would have been some legal precedent for this decision in the similar cases of Rodas and Putzer. However, as the physician charged with his care, it would have been difficult emotionally to allow him to die in this way. As his caregiver for several months, naturally I would have become attached to him emotionally. I would have had to use my conviction of the correctness of permitting him to die to overrule my personal emotional resistance to his decision.

Notes

1. A. Dumas, *The Count of Monte Cristo* (New York: E. P. Dutton, 1909), 2:43.

2. F. Plum and J. B. Posner, *The Diagnosis of Stupor and Coma* (Philadelphia: F. A. Davis, 1966).

3. R. E. Nordgren, W. R. Markesbery, and A. G. Reeves, "Seven Cases of Cerebromedullospinal Disconnection: The 'Locked-in' Syndrome," *Neurology* 21 (1971): 1140–48.

4. C. H. Hawkes and L. Bryan-Smyth, "The Electroencephalogram in the 'Locked-in' Syndrome, *Neurology* 24 (1974): 1015–18.

5. E. A. McCusker, R. A. Rudick, G. W. Honch, and R. C. Griggs, "Recovery from the Locked-in Syndrome," *Archives of Neurology* 39 (1982): 145–147.

6. M. H. Feldman, "Physiological Observations in a Chronic Case of Locked-in Syndrome, *Neurology* 21 (1971): 459–78.

7. G. E. Steffen and C. Franklin, "Who Speaks for the Patient with the Locked-in Syndrome?" *Hastings Center Report* 15(6) (1985): 13–15.

8. R. E. Cranford and D. R. Smith, "Consciousness: The Most Critical Moral (Constitutional) Standard for Human Personhood," *American Journal of Law and Medicine* 13 (1987): 233–48.

9. In re Rodas, No. 86PR139 (Colo Dist Ct Mesa Cty, Jan 22, 1987, *as modified*, April 3, 1987).

10. In the Matter of Murray Putzer, No. P–21–87E (Sup Ct NJ Chanc Div, July 9, 1987).

*This is a complex and sensitively described case that
reveals as much about the problems many doctors have in
dealing with dying patients as it does about the feisty
woman who is its subject. Stuart Youngner's description of
his involvement in the case is followed by a parallel description of the same events written by the patient's daughter.*

"I've Changed My Mind"

Stuart J. Youngner, M.D.

I WAS asked to consult in this case at the request of Dr. Ault, a busy
internist specializing in pulmonary diseases. He telephone me to
tell me about his patient, Mrs. Beach, briefly describing her medical situation and the reason he wanted me involved.

Mrs. Beach was a seventy-three-year-old widow who had suffered
for several years from chronic obstructive lung disease (COPD). Over
the past two years she had become progressively debilitated. Her difficulty in breathing was a constant source of discomfort and anxiety.
Treatment had required large doses of steroids, with unfortunate,
though entirely predictable, side effects. The first was bilateral cataracts that made reading, one of her few remaining pleasures, nearly
impossible. The second was osteoporosis, a thinning and weakening
of the structure of her bones, which led, in turn, to the collapse of several vertebrae and the fracture of ribs. Any attempt to halt or even
reduce the steroids resulted in the deterioration of her pulmonary
condition.

Because of these problems she had been admitted to the hospital

Stuart Youngner is Associate Professor of Psychiatry, Medicine, and Biomedical
Ethics at Case Western Reserve School of Medicine.

several times in the past year, including three stays in the medical intensive care unit. She had suffered a great deal.

"She says she's ready to die," said Dr. Ault. "She wants me to admit her to the hospital, stop all of her medications, and keep her comfortable while she dies." I had worked with Dr. Ault on several occasions and knew him to be an intelligent and thorough physician who was not unwilling to stop life-sustaining treatment at the request of patients whose quality of life had become unacceptable to them. In fact, during her last hospitalizations he had agreed to Mrs. Beach's request not to be resuscitated in the event of a cardiac arrest.

"This case is different," he said. "She is not terminal. She could die within the month, but she might well live for another two years. I feel uncomfortable bringing a relatively stable patient into the hospital with the sole purpose of withholding medication and letting her die. It seems too active somehow. Furthermore, I think she is quite manipulative—when she says she wants to die, I'm not sure she means it. If she means it, why doesn't she stop taking the medication and die at home? Why involve others? Moreover, she's gotten hold of literature from right-to-die groups."

I agreed to see Mrs. Beach in consultation; she called me later that day for an appointment, which we scheduled for early the next week.

I found her alone in my waiting room, seated in a wheelchair. She asked if I would push her to my office, but when we got there, she stood and insisted on walking in under her own power.

She was a tall, slim, well-dressed woman with a twinkle in her eye. She seemed both dignified and anxious to please, a seeming paradox that I never entirely understood. She immediately impressed me as bright and articulate. She moved with obvious difficulty, and each change of position (for example, going from a standing to sitting position or vice versa) caused her considerable pain. Her breathing was labored, but she seemed more comfortable as the interview proceeded.

She thanked me for seeing her so promptly and told me that she had inquired about me from several contacts at the university and had indeed read some of my publications. My credentials as a patients' rights advocate were in order, and she was hopeful that I could be of assistance to her. Mrs. Beach then filled in the details about her illness and her wish to die.

She had been fiercely independent, had enjoyed her life, and had worked hard to make the most of it. Twenty-nine years earlier, her husband had died suddenly in his sleep, from a heart attack. She was left alone to raise two teenage daughters. When they left home she went to work as a secretary in one of the university's professional schools. When she retired at sixty-five, she was administrative assistant to the chairman of the department.

She was proud of her accomplishments, both at work and in raising her two daughters, with whom she remained close despite the fact that they lived out of town. She was closest to Phyllis, the youngest, who had made many trips to Cleveland over the past year to help support and care for her mother.

Mrs. Beach had many close friends. A Wednesday night canasta club of many years' duration still continued at her apartment, despite the fact that she was usually too ill and tired to join the game. Two friends brought in dinner every Monday evening. A maid came in to clean once a week, and the patient's sister came every day to shop, cook, and run errands, including driving the patient to her numerous doctors' appointments. The patient appreciated this attention and affection but saw herself as dependent and nonproductive.

"My friends work or do something worthwhile," she complained. "I just live vicariously."

She spent many hours listening to classical music and said that it helped her to relax. She could no longer read much, however, because of the cataracts.

"They told me they can operate on my eyes, but what for?" she said. "They can't tell me how long I have to live. Besides, I've had enough with doctors and hospitals."

She described the anguish of her life over the past year. She was in constant pain from the fractured ribs and vertebrae. She could no longer cook for herself or clean the apartment.

"There is really no part of my body that doesn't hurt if you push it a bit too hard," she lamented. "And there is the agony of not being able to breathe without difficulty. Sometimes it feels like I'm drowning. It isn't exactly pain, but it is a terrible feeling. I use all my energy just to breathe. I don't want to be an invalid. I struggle every day not to be helpless. It takes me a half hour each morning to get up the nerve to get out of bed. I do it despite the pain. But I'm so tired of pushing."

The patient described her frequent hospitalizations and emergency room visits. She had been evaluated by the "pain team" at the hospital but had found no relief in a variety of medications and treatment with transcutaneous electrical nerve stimulation (TENS). She was helped by a series of ten nerve blocks, a procedure performed by an anesthe-siologist.

During the last of these procedures, in which an anesthetic is in-jected into a nerve near the site of the pain, one of her lungs was accidentally punctured and collapsed. The recommended treatment was insertion of a tube through her chest wall to reinflate the collapsed lung. Her daughter Phyllis flew in to be by her side. As in other recent admissions, a do-not-resuscitate (DNR) order was written, but the question of whether or not to insert the tube remained. The patient initially refused the tube, saying that she just wanted to die.

However, her physicians said that dying from the collapsed lung would be an extremely painful process. Phyllis talked the patient into accepting the chest tube. After a prolonged recovery, she was able to leave the hospital, but because of increased disability she sold her car. Another tangible symbol of her independence was gone.

The patient had been unsuccessfully treated for pain with a number of nonnarcotic analgesic and anti-inflammatory drugs. Most recently, she had consulted an orthopedic surgeon, who prescribed Demerol®, a potent synthetic narcotic, at the dose of fifty milligrams four times a day by mouth. Unfortunately, at this dose and by the oral route, Dem-erol is probably less potent than common aspirin. Her internist for many years, Dr. Calley, was reluctant to use more effective doses of narcotics, according to the patient, because such doses might further compromise her already delicate respiratory equilibrium.

The patient described how her father had died in a nursing home after a long illness. When the patient visited, he pled with her repeat-edly to let him die, that he did not "want to go on this way." Her older sister, Mary, had never married, and, according to the patient, devoted much of her life to caring for their ailing parents.

"What a waste. She constantly hovered over Dad, and now she's hovering over me. It's fine, I guess. I appreciate what she's doing, but I resent being the helpless one."

Mrs. Beach's disdain for helplessness was a dominant theme in our conversations. A second was her tremendous fear of pain, suffering, and death. She saw herself as weak and vulnerable in this regard.

"I can't stand pain," she told me. "I'm afraid it will get worse." At this point, and for the first time in my presence, she dissolved into tears. "It's so awful. Sometimes, when I'm alone, I cry out 'Oh God! Please let this be the end. Please take me away.' "

She quickly regained her composure. "I'm basically a coward. I hate to suffer."

Over the past six to eight months she had begun to think about doing something to end her life, either passively, by refusing treatment, or actively, by taking an overdose of medicine.

She cautiously informed me that she had literature from the Hemlock Society, an organization that openly endorses active euthanasia in hopelessly suffering patients and tells people how to take matters into their own hands "if their physicians refuse to cooperate." While Mrs. Beach spoke, she watched me intently, I believe she was trying to see how I was reacting (I didn't). She had saved up pills—enough, according to the Hemlock Society, to kill herself. The plan would be to take these pills and then put a plastic bag over her head. (At the suggestion of this grisly possibility, I winced.)

She was terribly frightened to try this, she confessed, out of anxiety not only that it would fail but that it would leave her in a more disabled state as well.

"Or maybe it would be a painful death," she said, "of which I would be aware and all alone. What if I threw up the pills and choked on my own vomit? There, you see, I *am* a coward."

Phyllis had offered to be with her mother if she chose this course, but Mrs. Beach had refused. "I wouldn't want to put my daughter through such a thing. Besides, she could get in trouble with the law."

"You know," she added, "if I knew *when* I was going to die, I think I could tough it out. It's the uncertainty that gets to me."

Although the pulmonary specialist, Dr. Ault, managed her acute care in the hospital, she was still followed by Dr. Calley, her internist. She liked Dr. Calley very much but thought he was uncomfortable talking about her wish to give up and die. Some months previously she had taken a list of the names and dosages of drugs she had saved up and asked him if they would be sufficient to end her life. According to the patient, he told her that if she took those drugs she would end up in worse shape than she was already in.

She felt frightened and isolated from her physicians. Dr. Calley clearly did not want to deal with her dilemma. Dr. Ault was immediately available for acute medical problems but had "neither the time nor inclination" to talk with her about her struggle. When she had pressed him, he referred her to me.

At the end of our first visit, I felt sympathetic to Mrs. Beach and the awful choices she faced. I did not see her as manipulative but rather as an effective advocate for herself in a system that had been somewhat unresponsive.

Her mind was clear and her power of reasoning excellent. There was no question of incompetence or lack of decision-making capacity. I did not think she was in the grip of a pathological depression. Her judgments seemed well reasoned and authentic to her particular personality and life experiences. In such circumstances, the desire to die can be quite rational.

In evaluating a wish to die in such patients, one should keep in mind two important caveats. First, the primary wish is rarely to die. If a medical intervention could restore an acceptable quality of life, patients like Mrs. Beach would not choose death. Unfortunately, the choice of getting better is not available. Death is merely the least worst alternative.

Second, patients who choose death may be frightened and ambivalent about their choice. For example, Mrs. Beach's fear of taking pills alone at home cannot be taken as proof that she did not "really" want to die. Such a conclusion would overlook or misrepresent how people actually make important decisions. In the important areas of our lives— marriage, divorce, friendship and career—we are usually quite discriminating and often fussy about particulars. We may have frequent misgivings and may even change our minds.

Should a choice about dying be any different? Certainly, it is a final decision, and as such it should be carefully thought through and examined—there is no room for impulsive trips to Las Vegas to die. But once thought through and examined, a choice to die need not be made in a totally unambivalent and undiscriminating manner.

I was not, however, ready to conclude that Mrs. Beach wanted to give up the struggle yet or that all had been done to nurture her will to live. It was clear that she felt isolated from and misunderstood by her physicians. But was it her wish to die or her wish for more control to which they were not adequately responding? I had seen patients in similar situations back off from a wish to die when pain was better controlled or communication with physicians was improved.

We scheduled a second appointment, and Mrs. Beach gave me permission to call her daughter Phyllis and her internist, Dr. Calley. I needed more information.

Phyllis was obviously glad I had called. She said her mother was pleased with our first visit.

"You're the first person who has listened to her. She felt so much better after talking with you."

Phyllis was an articulate, take-charge sort of person, much more adversarial and more obviously angry than her mother, of whom she was quite protective. She rejected out of hand the notion that her mother was manipulative or a complainer.

"She never even told us how sick she was until she couldn't hide it anymore." Phyllis confirmed her mother's independent spirit and fear of invalid status. She said her mother had always been a positive person, who had become increasingly unwilling to continue her current decline into utter helplessness.

"She's terribly afraid of pain," Phyllis confirmed. "In fact, she's almost preoccupied with it."

Phyllis had helped her mother draw up a Living Will and had been designated as her mother's proxy decision maker in the event her mother became "incompetent." She was aware of Mrs. Beach's efforts to collect a lethal dose of medication and told me she was willing to be there if and when her mother decided to take that step. However, it was clear that she was uncomfortable with that prospect, perhaps even a bit terrified.

She accepted my suggestion that better pain control and communication with physicians might diminish Mrs. Beach's preoccupation with dying, and she was supportive of any efforts I could make in that regard. She assured me that she would come to Cleveland whenever I asked. (I might add that Phyllis and her husband managed a successful business; she had significant responsibilities at home.)

I phoned Dr. Calley with some trepidation. He was a well-respected and successful internist, but I had always had the feeling that he was somewhat skeptical of the role psychiatry or medical ethics could play in the "real world" of medical practice.

He was uncomfortable with my call. He probably assumed I was going to try to persuade him to let Mrs. Beach die. He saw the patient as "somewhat manipulative and hysterical," and he had obviously been thrown off balance when she had consulted him about her "suicide plan." He wanted nothing to do with "killing her."

I assured him that I did not want him or anyone else to kill Mrs. Beach but was merely trying to collect information in order to assist Dr. Ault, who had "involved" me. I added that I also hoped to help the patient herself through difficult times. He became less defensive and agreed that she had had a difficult course, but he insisted that "her pain is not that bad, and she is not terminal." However, he agreed that fifty milligrams of Demerol by mouth was "probably not enough." He said he would be happy to write a prescription for a more effective drug.

Since he could not, by law, phone in the narcotics prescription, and it seemed unnecessary to send the patient's older sister out to Dr. Calley's office to pick it up, we agreed that I would write the prescription when I saw the patient the next day.

I told Mrs. Beach about Dr. Calley's willingness to give her a more effective painkiller and asked if she was willing to try it. She thought for a while and said she was.

"Frankly," she said, "I don't think my quality of life is acceptable even without the pain. I'm just going to get worse, with more broken bones and more painful medical procedures. But let's give it a try. Who knows, it might work."

She then brought up a variety of concerns: Would the new drug make her sick to her stomach? Would it make her too drowsy? I told here these were possibilities, but we would not know for sure unless we tried. She agreed to take the medication as prescribed and assured me that she would not overdose with it. I wrote the prescription for the short-acting narcotic suggested by Dr. Calley. I felt somewhat uncomfortable writing it, not because I feared Mrs. Beach would use it to end her life but because it moved me from the role of consultant to treating physician in an area outside my field of expertise.

I said good-bye to Mrs. Beach and made an appointment to see her in a week. I told her to keep in touch with me by phone to adjust the dose of medication. I then called Dr. Ault to check out my plan with him. He was quite agreeable and more than happy for me to manage her pain. "It's a sad irony," he commented, "that she has an internist, an orthopedic surgeon, and a pulmonologist, and it's the psychiatrist who ends up treating the pain."

Two days later the patient called. She sounded like a new person. There was more strength in her voice. She was almost euphoric.

"The medication is working wonders," she told me. "I don't want to die. I have more energy and a positive outlook. I can get around much better. Thank you so much."

Of course, it was too good to be true. The next day she called to tell me that the medication was no longer "holding." It seemed to wear off after three hours (she was taking it every four hours as needed). I suggested taking the medication every three hours and, if that did not work, doubling the dose. She called the next day to tell me she was feeling too drowsy and "spaced-out."

"I don't like the feeling of having to take more and more medicine. It makes me feel like I'm losing control," she complained.

When I next saw her, she was definitely discouraged. She complained of severe pain in her back and difficulty in breathing. She had tried various methods of adjusting the medication but to no avail. It either did not work or made her sleepy. I realized that she was becoming habituated to the pain-relieving effects of the drug but seemed unable to tolerate the increase necessary to control her pain. The patient was asking again that we examine the option of admitting her to the hospital to let her die.

When I discussed this with Dr. Ault, he suggested that we bring the issue before the hospital's ethics committee, which met at the request of clinicians, patients, or families and gave advice. It did not make decisions. The committee had functioned for over ten years and had heard many cases. Its members were a thoughtful, considerate group with a great deal of experience, though none so far with a case just like this one. I had been serving as chairman of the committee for some five years.

Dr. Ault and I agreed that it might be helpful to have the committee hear and discuss the issues before a crisis developed. This would also give the patient and perhaps Phyllis a chance to talk with the committee members directly and present their case. Dr. Ault said he would be more receptive to carrying out Mrs. Beach's request if the committee thought it was reasonable.

The support of a hospital ethics committee can be perceived by a physician as helpful in at least two ways. First, it may furnish evidence that his or her own decision is not deviant or idiosyncratic but is shared by a group of respected peers. Second, it may offer legal protection: the success of any future legal action against the physician would be lessened if an ethics committee had corroborated the decision.

Mrs. Beach and Phyllis agreed. Both were enthusiastic about talking with the committee, so I scheduled a meeting for the following week. I also told the patient I was not comfortable managing her pain and wanted to involve someone with more expertise (and confidence). She agreed that I would attend to it when I got back to town; I was to be at a meeting in Washington, D.C., for two days.

When I returned, I found the patient had been hospitalized. She had further injured her back, and her sister had taken her to see Dr. Ault, who judged the pain severe enough to require hospital admission. Phyllis and her husband had arrived from out of town and were at the patient's side.

Mrs. Beach was curled up in bed in obvious discomfort. She was quite alert, however, and glad to see me. An initial effort to control her pain with morphine had been a "fiasco." The patient was allergic to morphine. She experienced severe nausea and broke out in a bothersome rash. A pain expert had been called in, and Mrs. Beach was switched to a long-acting analgesic, methadone, supplemented with a short-acting one, Dilaudid®. I felt some relief that pain control was no longer my responsibility.

Initially, Mrs. Beach and Phyllis were hopeful that the pain could be controlled and that the patient could return to her apartment. Both, however, wanted to keep the meeting with the ethics committee, now six days away.

I visited the patient and her daughter daily. Phyllis was an aggressive advocate for her mother. She was an informed consumer who asked many questions and expected answers rather than platitudes. From my point of view she was never inappropriate in her efforts to secure the best care possible, both technical and humane, for her mother.

The human aspect of care does not always come easily or consistently in a large academic medical center, with multiple consultants, attending physicians, residents, and students coming and going as various rotations change or physicians "cover" for each other on evenings and weekends. For patients like Mrs. Beach, the goals of technical care and hospitalization shift to comfort rather than cure. In these circumstances the quality of the interaction with health professionals becomes a matter of primary rather than secondary concern. To be treated with respect and dignity, to be listened to, communicated with, and recognized as a unique individual, are qualities of care too often lacking in the complex, impersonal setting of a modern hospital. Mrs. Beach and, increasingly, her daughter, as Mrs. Beach became weaker, did not accept this setting passively.

For some health professionals involved in their care, Mrs. Beach and Phyllis became irritants. The word spread quickly that the patient's predicament was unusual—she was considering stopping her breathing medications and dying right on *their* ward, perhaps even on their shift. The patient and her daughter were constantly asking questions: What dose of Dilaudid was she receiving? When would she get the next dose of methadone? What had the pain consultant written in the chart? Where was Dr. Ault? When would he be by that day?

The patient's care became more complicated as she either experienced unacceptable levels of pain or was rendered nearly stuporous from increased doses of narcotics. She remained fearful and worried that she would only become more helpless and dependent.

My job, aside from comforting the mother and daughter, was to function as liaison and communicator between the various health professionals. I attempted to clarify contradictory statements, to translate technical information, and to get calls through to important decision makers when Mrs. Beach and Phyllis could not. I tried to help everyone focus on specific goals as a means of facilitating decision making. I made sure that the night or weekend shifts were up to date on how and when pain medication would be given; too often small but important details are lost at such times. Occasionally, I soothed egos bruised by open criticism or, more often, sarcastic comments.

In a sense I had taken on the role of mediator or communications broker. Is this role a reasonable one for an ethics consultant? I believe so. So often the ethical problems in a given case are aggravated or even created by communications difficulties, misperceptions, and personality clashes. An ethics consultant who is not aware of or ignores such issues will often be ineffective.

At times I found myself reacting with impatience. Was I being manipulated by this pair of women whom we could so rarely satisfy? Was the current situation indeed *their* fault?

Of course, it was no one's fault, just a miserable illness in a technological setting that had little to offer this proud and independent woman, brought now to the verge of despair. She had struggled valiantly, I reminded myself. Was it too much to ask us to understand and accommodate her "fussiness" in the face of so much uncertainty and suffering? Was Phyllis acting inappropriately, or was she acting exactly as any of us would wish our daughter, spouse, or parent to act if we were helpless in such a frightening place as a modern hospital?

I tried to help some staff members overcome their resentment and irritations by sharing some of the thinking I had used to overcome my own worst instincts. I feared lest the staff's discomfort be translated into decreased communication, further isolating the patient and her daughter at the hour they most needed understanding and support. One incident in particular is quite poignant in this regard.

Dr. Riley was the first-year resident responsible for Mrs. Beach's care.

Dr. Ault came once a day, but Dr. Riley was on the ward at all times. He performed a variety of small but important tasks in her daily care. Dr. Ault's plans were conveyed to Dr. Riley via phone calls, written notes in the chart, or directly if Dr. Riley was not tied up with something more urgent (he often was) when Dr. Ault showed up on the ward. Unlike some private and most staff cases, Dr. Riley did not have a primary or even a shared decision-making role in Mrs. Beach's care. Yet he was there to do most of the work.

I had come to know Dr. Riley at least superficially as our paths crossed in the care of other patients. He had always seemed a sensitive, bright, and committed young physician. One day as I was talking with Phyllis, I asked how things were going with Dr. Riley.

She scowled. "He won't give us the time of day," she complained. "On morning rounds he barely sticks his head in the door. He takes ages to come when the nurse calls him, and when he does show up, he's curt and seems put out." I was puzzled.

The next day I was sitting at the nurses' station writing a note in the chart. In the next room a group of residents and medical students were talking. Dr. Riley was complaining bitterly.

"You can't believe it," I overheard him say. "They admitted this lady to the hospital to help her die! That's not why I became a doctor. Can you believe it? They are considering stopping her medicine and letting her die. It's wrong. Besides, I'm just a flunky. Why should I have to participate? I could even get into legal trouble."

I felt I should say something but felt like an intruder. "Do you mind if I join your discussion?" I asked, overcoming my own discomfort. No one objected, so I stepped through the door and sat down. "It sounds like you all have some real concerns about this case," I began. "Have you had a chance to discuss them with Dr. Ault or your attending physician [the faculty member directly responsible for supervising the residents' work]?"

No one had. It was mid-July. Two weeks earlier, Dr. Riley had been a medical student! And yet, in the rush to complete all of the physical examinations, order the lab tests, read x rays and CAT scans, and juggle mounds of data, no one had had the time to help this twenty-five-year-old physician of two weeks experience with the awesome responsibility of caring for a patient like Mrs. Beach. No wonder he was angry.

I explained to the group the history of the case and my work with Mrs. Beach and Phyllis. I reviewed with them briefly the social and legal consensus over the past two decades which recognized the right of competent patients to refuse even life-sustaining treatment.

"There is no legal danger here, in my opinion," I said, "but your moral discomfort seems quite reasonable. Other physicians and a segment of society probably share that discomfort. If you feel strongly, it would be entirely reasonable and proper for you to request not to be involved in Mrs. Beach's care. In fact, if you think it would be helpful, I'd be happy to talk with your attending physician or Dr. Ault."

One resident said she thought Mrs. Beach's request was quite reasonable. A medical student added her opinion that the patient had suffered enough and that we had an obligation to support her wishes. I told them that the ethics committee was meeting in two days, and all were welcome to participate. I told Dr. Riley that his views, in particular, would be quite helpful in framing the discussion. I chose not to say anything to Dr. Riley then or in private about Phyllis's comments.

The next day Phyllis greeted me at the door to her mother's room. "What did you say to Dr. Riley?" she asked. "He's changed completely. He couldn't be more considerate or helpful. He comes right away. He goes out of his way to make Mom feel comfortable. He told me he didn't agree with any decision to stop treatment, but he respected our wishes."

I was not surprised. Physicians, not unlike patients, prefer to feel in control of, or at least informed about, what is going on around them. Too often residents and nurses must take a major responsibility in carrying out plans, about which they have had little input. As in the case of Mrs. Beach, such decisions are often the choice between the lesser of two evils. The decision makers often help resolve their ambivalence about such decisions by making them. There is no such help for those who are handed decisions without participating in them. Such persons often feel resentful, used, and oppositional. It seemed that, like Mrs. Beach, Dr. Riley felt better when someone listened to him.

Things were not going well for Mrs. Beach. Her caregivers could not strike a balance between keeping her alert and keeping her pain under control. Not surprisingly, her hope dimmed, and her wish to discontinue her breathing medications came to the fore. She appeared to be very tired and had withdrawn from social and emotional interaction with those around her. The nursing staff, particularly her primary nurse, were very supportive and close to the patient and her daughter. They were quite comfortable with stopping treatment.

Two days before the ethics committee was to meet, the patient asked that her steroids and other breathing medication be stopped. Dr. Ault was convinced that the patient had suffered enough and that her wishes should be honored. He wrote an order to that effect. "I still want the committee to meet," he told me, "but I cannot in good conscience force her to take this medication."

She had already taken her dose of steroids that day but had not received any when I saw her the following day. She looked very frail and was lying on her side straining to breathe. "No more medicine. No more suffering," she gasped. I held her hand and asked her if there was anything more I could do.

"No more pain. No more pain," she repeated over and over again.

"You are very brave," I told her. She shook her head from side to side. "No," she whispered, "I'm a coward." She closed her eyes and nodded her assent when I asked if she wanted to stop talking.

Mrs. Beach's relatives were called in from out of town. Along with the in-town family, they came to her room to say their good-byes. Phyllis was always by her side, sleeping next to her mother at night in an easy chair. The ethics committee was scheduled to meet the next day. Phyllis would attend alone; Mrs. Beach was too ill. I invited Mrs. Beach's nurses and called to invite Dr. Calley, who sounded uncomfortable but said he'd try to be there.

The next morning at three o'clock, Mrs. Beach woke Phyllis.

"What is it, Mom?" she asked.

"I don't want to die," said Mrs. Beach. "I've changed my mind."

Later that morning she told Dr. Ault the same thing. We were all taken by surprise. When I saw the patient at noon, she was in severe discomfort. Earlier in the day she had refused her pain medication. She kept her eyes closed. When I tried to discuss her change of heart, she was so weak I could barely hear her.

"I'm too tired. No more pain. I don't want the pain medicine," she told me enigmatically.

I was, like everyone else, confused and dismayed. The patient seemed more withdrawn than ever, and it was very difficult for me to determine her level of decision-making capacity, let alone interpret her contradictory requests.

That afternoon the ethics committee met. Phyllis was agreeable to the format: the committee would meet alone both before and after her appearance. She was quite anxious, as was I. I felt somewhat foolish. Was Dr. Calley correct that the patient was "manipulative"? Had I been manipulated? How was the committee going to react to all of this?

Because I saw myself primarily as an advocate for Mrs. Beach, I stepped down as chair of the meeting, turning those duties over to my co-chair, a nurse who was actually one of the committee's founders. A dozen committee members came. In addition to Phyllis, guests included one of Mrs. Beach's nurses and Dr. Ault. Mrs. Beach's resident, Dr. Riley, and Dr. Calley did not attend. The meeting began with a presentation of the case. Dr. Ault covered the medical history, and I filled in the details of my work with the patient.

When Phyllis came in, she was initially quite anxious. The warm interest of committee members quickly put her at ease. The chairperson reiterated that the committee functioned only as an advisory body, in this case to Dr. Ault, her mother, and herself. Phyllis explained her belief that Mrs. Beach's overriding wish was to stop the medication and be allowed to die as comfortably as possible. She thought the wish had been well considered and was consistent with her mother's previous values and preferences. Phyllis cried openly at several points during the discussion. Committee members were sympathetic and supportive. At various points they asked for clarifications, and their questions were always polite but quite pointed and helpful in clarifying the issues.

Phyllis and I both tried to explain the recent change of heart. We agreed that Mrs. Beach had clearly revoked her wish to stop taking medicine and die. We were less certain why. Perhaps she had looked death in the face and blinked. Unfortunately, she was so weak and withdrawn that it was difficult, if not impossible, to explore her reasoning in any depth.

We were convinced that Mrs. Beach did not want to endure further pain and suffering. How this could be accomplished was less clear. How long could we keep her in the hospital? Could she be managed at home? Phyllis said she was willing to try to arrange this but was apprehensive about caring for her in her apartment—Mrs. Beach was quite ill and had been getting large doses of pain medication. A nursing home would be anathema to her. If she went home and decided again that she wanted to die, would the hospital take her back? No alternatives seemed reasonable or obvious.

The committee members were neither shocked nor irritated by Mrs. Beach's apparent ambivalence. They did nothing to make Dr. Ault, Phyllis, or myself feel foolish. They communicated a real sense of understanding and acceptance.

When Phyllis left the room, the discussion focused on the patient's need to be in control. The committee members saw this need as an important and legitimate part of her character and felt it should be supported and honored, whether being in control meant taking the medication or refusing it. In other words, if the patient again changed her mind and refused the medication, we should not force it on her. Their opinion was influenced to a great degree by Phyllis's obvious knowledge of and devotion to her mother. It was also clear, from various perspectives, that the patient was suffering a great deal and would only get worse with time.

The committee said there was no need to rush Mrs. Beach out of the hospital and suggested that we take a few days to let things "settle" while we continued to discuss and evaluate her wishes. Following the meeting, I discussed these recommendations with Phyllis, who was relieved and said she found the meeting very affirming.

Mrs. Beach did change her mind that day—again by refusing the steroids on numerous occasions. She regularly accepted the pain medications. Off the steroids, her breathing steadily deteriorated. Four days after the ethics committee meeting she died.

I learned a great deal from my contact with Mrs. Beach, Phyllis, and the various health professionals involved in the case. It illustrated the vital importance of communication and understanding when medical technology has little to offer. How difficult it is for strangers, thrown together by fate, to negotiate the awesome responsibility of giving up and letting go. I believe my involvement in those negotiations was helpful.

The ethics committee was helpful, too. I am convinced that the mere awareness of its availability was reassuring to a number of us. The meeting itself offered tangible help via clarification, support, and affirmation that the values and concerns of this dying woman and her daughter were reasonable and proper. Helping them was an appropriate role for physicians and nurses.

Exactly what went on in Mrs. Beach's mind those last few days remains something of a mystery. My best guess is that her wish to die had been doubly motivated: first, by a desire to escape the torment that had become her life and, second, by a need to regain the control that had steadily slipped away. She regained some control when the system finally said yes to her treatment refusal. But when there was nothing between her and the death she had pursued, its newly felt reality frightened her, and she paused to reconsider. We allowed her this, and when it became clear that torment remained the only other alternative, she chose to die.

The Patient's Daughter

My mother died on July 11, 1988. Some might say that her death at seventy-three was premature; she would have argued that her death was long overdue. She was not only my mother; she was my friend. The following is my experience of the long road she traveled to find support for her wish to die.

Illness was never a focal point in our home. Although Mom was diagnosed with emphysema when she was in her forties, neither her emphysema nor her other physical ailments merited more from her than a statement of the problem and the proposed solution. She was not a complainer. She dealt with physical and emotional pain by going into her room and lying down until she felt better.

Her life was a direct reflection of her personality. She had lived alone for the last twenty-five years and had created a life-style that supported her fierce independence and need for privacy as well as her great enjoyment of friends and family. Although she was highly opinionated and strong-willed, she was also very interested in and loyal to others. Reading was an important part of my mother's life, but she'd drop any book for a good canasta game or dinner with friends. I could always count on her for a heated political discussion, the intricacies of a new recipe, or a good laugh (she had a great sense of humor).

Although the effects of emphysema took their toll steadily, Mom didn't quit smoking until a few years before she died. I don't know if that's a testament to the addiction or to her stubbornness! Physically, she carried on with no expectation of special treatment. Her life-style didn't really change—it just slowed down. Mom didn't want to draw attention to herself, so she'd often push herself beyond reason, only to pay for it soon after with significant breathing difficulty. She was tall and thin, and she carried herself well, so it was easy to see when she was in trouble. If anyone voiced a concern, however, she'd shrug it off and point out that this was part and parcel of the disease. Mom constantly asked us not to worry—she was fine.

She wasn't fine, but she did appear to have adjusted to living with a chronic illness. I adjusted with her. In retrospect I can now see that for many years she was dealing with numerous and extensive medical problems. For some reason, I never actually perceived her as someone who was ill.

Her relationships with physicians seemed to be based on a traditional paternalistic medical model. She was extremely trusting of her doctors, even those she did not particularly like. For someone who believed so strongly in her ability to make autonomous decisions, my mother was uncharacteristically willing to relinquish her power to members of the medical profession.

Mom's operational belief was that she could take care of herself. She rarely requested assistance from anyone, and she specifically requested that neither my sister nor I speak with her doctors without her permission. Not only was it important for her to be in control, she also feared that we might upset the apple cart. She felt that pleasant, obedient behavior would produce the best care. Any intervention on our part would be construed as interference with her long-established model of medical conduct.

In January 1987, my mother's carefully constructed walls of independence began to crumble. She was hospitalized twice that month; each time she was released as soon as the results from her pulmonary tests and blood gases fell within some predetermined range.

When I spoke with her the morning of her second release, the weakness and depression in her voice convinced me that I needed to be with her. Like a well-trained daughter, I asked her if she'd mind if I came to her. Her only response was "Thank you, but I don't want to put you to any trouble." I was on the next plane to Cleveland.

Nothing could have prepared me for the next few months. When I arrived at her apartment, Mom was lying in bed with tears rolling down her face. She didn't know what was wrong with her. She was experiencing extreme pain in her hip and side when she lay still and even worse pain when she moved. Her breathing was frighteningly shallow. The bathroom was about ten feet from her bed, and it took every ounce of her energy to get there. She refused to consider a bed pan. Getting into position to take medications or breathing treatments required planning and patience. I had never seen her like this. More important, she had never before felt like this.

Mom had no idea about her prognosis. She only knew that Dr. Ault, her pulmonary specialist, had told her that she was well enough to go home. Nobody in the hospital thought to ask her if she'd have any help at home; they just sent her on her way. Mom knew before she left the hospital that she was too weak to care for herself, yet she said nothing to Dr. Ault or to any of the staff.

That day she began talking with me about wanting to die. I think that what kicked off her previously dormant thoughts about death was her constant pain, along with the realization that she now needed to rely on others. As if her current problems weren't enough to deal with, Mom was also questioning the potential problems that might arise from the high doses of steroid medication she was now taking.

Mom was very sick and in great pain, and we were both frightened. We agreed that, for now, she was too ill to make any decisions. So, although I was always conscious of her need for autonomy, I began to take over. It was the beginning of an emotionally devastating time for both of us. All I wanted to do was make her better, but I didn't know how, and her doctors turned out to be of no help.

I phoned her two primary physicians, Dr. Ault and Dr. Calley, a general internist. From those initial conversations I learned that we had to ask specific questions to get the kind of information we needed. Unfortunately, it took me a long time to learn what the questions needed to be.

Dr. Ault insisted that Mom's tests indicated that she should be basically all right. If she was having problems, they were probably due to anxiety which, he informed me, was a problem common to COPD patients. Mom had warned me ahead of time that Dr. Ault was a rather intimidating man, and our conversation did nothing to negate that description.

Dr. Calley, on the other hand, was warm and empathic after first pointing out that Dr. Ault was the doctor in charge and that I should speak with him. As for my mother's pain, the most he could do was recommend Tylenol® because "we don't want to compromise her breathing."

I didn't know where to turn for help. Mom needed twenty-four-hour care, which came from me, my sister, and nurse's aides. Aunt Mary, Mom's older sister, was on vacation in Florida at the time, and Mom was adamant about Aunt Mary's not coming home early. She did not want to have to be cared for by anyone, least of all by her sister, whom Mom felt had spent enough of her life caring for others.

Now Mom's focus was on wanting to die. She thought, however, that she might not feel so strongly about wanting to die if someone could tell her that it was just a matter of time before she could be relatively pain-free, reasonably mobile, and self-sufficient once again. She badly wanted to know what was in store for her, and her doctors either didn't know or didn't want to comment. I felt that if we could get some honest answers, we might be able to reassess both treatment and life goals.

Mom was not improving and was not willing to call Dr. Ault before her next scheduled appointment. This was typical of her: she didn't trust her ability to judge her need for help. She was afraid of being considered a hypochondriac and being told that the problem was all in her mind.

On the day of my mother's appointment with Dr. Ault, she and I contacted anyone I thought might be a potential resource in contributing to Mom's improvement. We met with a social worker who talked to my mother as if she were a three-year-old child. The only thing worse than watching Mom in pain was listening to her being condescended to by someone who should have known better.

We spent time with a nutritionist figuring out how to interest Mom in eating. We spent time with an occupational therapist trying to find some alternative possibilities for handling basic routines.

And we spent time with Dr. Ault. Our interactions with him were often frustrating—probably for him as well as for us. It was obvious that he was uncomfortable with emotional situations, and Mom and I were both in highly emotional states. His discomfort lessened when he was in control of a basically pragmatic discussion. Our very different styles of communication did not make for an easy relationship on any of our parts.

Mom's seventy-second birthday was February 15. I thought it would be her last. She had no interest in being alive. Her pain and the number of medications she was taking were playing havoc with her. She was aware of her inability to concentrate and her lack of interest in anything outside her physical condition. We were both overwhelmed by a sense of helplessness and hopelessness. My mother was not at all religious, and yet every day she asked God to please let her go to sleep and not wake up.

Right after her birthday, Mom fell in the bathroom. Her aide took her to the emergency room where x-ray readings found nothing wrong, so she went home. Two days later, the visiting nurse answered the phone when I called; they were waiting for an ambulance to arrive. Mom's breathing was very bad, and she was admitted to intensive care.

Carol, Mom's ICU nurse, told me when I called that Mom had informed the hospital that under no circumstances did she want CPR or any mechanical intervention to keep her alive. A psychologist showed up, presumably to ascertain competency for legal purposes. I guess Mom passed that hurdle, because a DNR order was entered on her record.

Carol was not overly optimistic about Mom's prognosis, so I got on the next plane. I got to the ICU in time to meet the anesthesiologist called in to administer a nerve block for Mom's pain. Someone had thought to reread the xrays taken the day of her fall and had discovered rib fractures on the side that hurt so badly. Nerve blocks seemed to be a logical, successful solution for the pain.

ICU beds are understandably kept open for people who want to stay alive. As a result, Mom was moved as soon as her condition stabilized. She was receiving steroids intravenously and nerve blocks on request. Although the blocks greatly relieved the pain, Mom worried about them being administered by interns or residents who might not have had enough sleep. Her pain diminished, however, and it looked as if a few days in the hospital might make a real difference in her recovery. We discussed her DNR request, which she felt more strongly about than ever. Mom was adamant that the pain she experienced from her breathing difficulty made death a welcome visitor. She indicated that if she was lucky enough to lose consciousness, she did not want to be revived. I promised to defend her request.

On the third morning, a needle from one of the nerve blocks punctured her lung. Watching her was like watching all of the air escape from a balloon. The only words she could manage were "I can't breathe; I want to die."

One of the emergency room physicians happened to be walking by the room as floor staff were running in. He wanted to insert a chest tube and began ordering the necessary supplies. I explained that Mom wanted to die and that I needed to know what the result would be of *not* inserting the tube. He suggested that without the tube she would continue to gasp for breath, then ultimately die from respiratory failure; she would get morphine for the pain, but she would probably suffer considerably. I advised Mom to have the tube inserted, and I held her hand while the physician pushed the tube through her chest, using no anesthesia. My mother never flinched.

When her breathing improved, Mom asked me why I didn't let her die. Although she didn't want to put up with anything else going wrong, I didn't see how I could stand back and watch her needlessly suffer. There did come a time, however, when I wished that I had had the courage to refuse the tube and let nature take its course.

The collapsed lung necessitated an extended hospital stay. Mom worked hard at presenting an optimistic spirit most of the time while regularly confiding to me that she still wished she had died. One of her nurses suggested that we request a floor conference with Dr. Ault to get some answers about what to expect. We requested the conference, but Dr. Ault seemed to minimize the concern; after all, as soon as Mom's lung healed, she would be much better and probably capable of returning to normal activity.

Surprisingly, her lung did heal, and Mom actually returned home with some renewed strength. Since the disaster from the nerve block, however, she was receiving no alternative method of pain relief. The pain seemed to concentrate on one side of her body, from her neck down to her hip, and began also to appear in her back. Neither Dr. Ault nor Dr. Calley considered her pain to be a problem that they needed to treat. As a matter of fact, Dr. Calley wrote off most of her pain as arthritis: take two Tylenol and *don't* call me in the morning!

Mom's return home in March 1987 necessitated a readjustment to living alone. She badly wanted to take over responsibility for herself once again, and we both felt that with regular visits from my aunt she would be all right. Every action was painful for her, but she managed to maintain herself and her apartment with help from family and friends. She rarely went out; my aunt did Mom's shopping, and friends regularly visited with dinner.

And still she talked about wanting to die with everyone near her. Material arrived regularly from the Hemlock Society, and I began reading everything I could on death and dying. I hoped that as long as we actually talked about the subject, Mom wouldn't actually *do* anything about committing suicide.

While she enjoyed some relatively good days, Mom became increasingly debilitated by her pain as well as distraught over the side effects from the steroids. Cataracts made reading slow and uncomfortable; rib fractures made sitting for any length of time a frustrating, painful endeavor; loss of strength in her hands and trembling in her fingers precluded her participation in meal preparation, which she loved, and made it extremely difficult for her to even open pill bottles.

Although at various times Mom questioned her physicians about the potential harm from the combinations and dosages of drugs, she never got more than a "there's not much we can do about it" response. She finally ordered the book *Worst Pills, Best Pills* and checked out each one of her medications. She became even more convinced that the treatment for the problems of emphysema was more life-denying than the disease. With the steroids, in particular, she was in a Catch-22 situation. Whenever the steroids were decreased, her breathing capacity diminished, and the pain she so badly wanted to avoid would return.

By the end of 1987, Mom had stockpiled enough combined medication to produce lethal results. She also signed her Living Will. During a weekend together, we went over the Living Will as well as the instructions for taking the pills if and when she really felt the time had come. Although she initially indicated that she wanted nobody present when she took the pills (she was afraid of involving another person), she wound up promising not to take them unless I was there. I was willing to sit in another room, but I wasn't willing to face the possibility of my mother struggling alone.

I never found our conversations maudlin. On the contrary, these talks were always interspersed with gossip, politics, news of her grandchildren, and giggles. Talking about death simply became an integral part of our lives.

In the spring of 1987, Mom reached a breaking point with the pain in her hip and surprised even herself by unceasingly complaining to Dr. Calley. He finally referred her to an orthopedist, who discovered calcium deposits in her hip and an overall lack of calcium in her body. She had actually hoped that she might get a diagnosis of terminal cancer! Instead, she got news of one more chronic problem: there was little chance that the fractures would heal and a significant probability of continuous new fractures. What Mom appreciated most about this doctor was the corroboration that her pain was real. He was the first physician to prescribe a painkiller stronger than Tylenol. The medication didn't work, though, and Mom was reluctant to phone back for help. She didn't want to bother him.

Eventually Mom decided that she would take the stockpiled pills if she could have some assurance directly from a trusted medical authority that the pills would work. She took her "prescription for suicide" to Dr. Calley and asked him to look over her list and tell her whether or not she had enough pills to produce death. As Mom described it, Dr. Calley became quite angry and informed her that not only would the pills *not* work, but she'd wind up in even worse shape if she took them.

She actually apologized for upsetting him, and to me she expressed the belief that Dr. Calley would not want to see her again. She felt badly that she had burdened him with her problem, but she was right—Mom never saw him again. Although Dr. Calley was not the admitting doctor in most of her hospitalizations, he had always stopped by each day to say hello. During her final stay in the hospital, Dr. Calley was conspicuous by his absence. He did achieve his purpose, however. He wanted no part in contributing to Mom's death, and she was now too petrified to consider taking the pills.

Mom then began to research other methods of suicide. One she thought might work was a combination of ingesting the pills and then loosely tying a plastic bag around her head. I persuaded her to continue her research!

In May 1988, Mom finally told Dr. Ault in words he could hear and understand that she'd had enough and she wanted to die. No matter how difficult I found communication with Dr. Ault, I will always be thankful to him for suggesting that Mom call Dr. Stuart Youngner.

Before scheduling an appointment with Stuart, Mom checked him out through a friend in the medical school. She received a thumbs-up review, along with a number of articles written by and about Dr. Youngner. She was actually looking forward to seeing him.

As a psychiatrist and the chairman of the hospital ethics committee, Stuart became a major support and advocate for my mother. In the six weeks prior to her death, Mom saw him or spoke with him regularly. At his request, and with my mother's concurrence, I spoke at length with Stuart following Mom's first visit with him. He actually invited my input! I had an overwhelming sense of relief after our conversation. Here was a member of a system I distrusted who could be trusted. Here was a person who stayed away from platitudes. Here was a doctor who was not threatened or frightened or angered by my mother's wish to die. From the start, Stuart acted as a guide whose respect for my mother empowered her beautifully. He agreed with her that her wish to die was not unreasonable, thereby allowing her to make room, albeit reluctantly, for one more helper.

Stuart immediately prescribed what he thought might be a more effective painkiller. He suggested the possibility that if her pain was controlled, Mom might not be so committed to dying. He also explained to us both that as she began to build up a tolerance for the painkillers, she would need higher and higher doses. The drugs did initially alleviate some of the pain, but Mom felt they affected her alertness. She would not take the pills unless she was desperate. Consequently, she wasn't ever able to get ahead of the pain.

Stuart felt that Mom would ultimately need support from Dr. Ault or Dr. Calley in carrying out her wishes. He spoke with both of them. Dr. Ault agreed that stopping her medications would bring about Mom's death, but he did not want her in the hospital under his care for that purpose. He had no problem with her stopping medication and dying at home. Dr. Calley, not surprisingly, preferred to let others handle the situation.

Mom wanted to die at home, but we all agreed that the hospital could provide the best access to pain control. At no time did any doctor give us assurance that Mom wouldn't suffer or be in pain, but I still believed that if the common goal was pain control, suffering would not be an issue.

Stuart then suggested that a meeting with the ethics committee might provide Dr. Ault with some moral support. If members of the committee advised that it would be appropriate for Mom to discontinue the treatment that was keeping her alive, then perhaps Dr. Ault would reconsider his position. Mom and I were invited to be present at the July 7 meeting.

On July 1, my aunt found my mother in such extraordinary pain that she insisted on taking her to Dr. Ault—who immediately admitted Mom for the specific purpose of pain control. Miracles can happen!

A pharmacologist monitored drugs and doses over a few days, and Mom wound up with a successful combination of Dilaudid and methadone. We had been warned about the probable need for higher doses to continue managing the pain, and that was exactly what happened. The floor resident made his position clear: he did not approve of the amount of medication Mom was getting. He felt that she would become addicted to the drugs and/or the drugs would cause her death. How could anyone in his right mind truly worry about addiction under these circumstances? I did not want Mom to get overmedicated. I did not want her to die. But I also did not want her to suffer. That was the only occasion where I expressly asked a doctor to stay away from my mother. That resident didn't enter her room again.

By July 6, Mom was alternately in some pain, in emotional withdrawal, and at times in what I perceived was a false sense of well-being. She was taking all her medications orally, with difficulty. When her nurse brought her steroid medication that morning, she told us very simply that she wanted to die. I asked her to take her medicine and promised to speak with Stuart and Dr. Ault to see what support we could count on.

Dr. Ault responded quickly to my call. He actually pointed out to me that he knew she had a right to refuse treatment and that he had a duty to not let her suffer. Without waiting for the ethics committee meeting, he would change the orders on Mom's chart to withhold her steroids. He visited Mom, who clearly repeated her wish to die, and Dr. Ault assured her that the staff would keep her as comfortable as possible.

Stuart saw Mom alone shortly thereafter and satisfied himself that

Mom was quite lucid in her thinking and speaking. He felt that one way he could support her was to talk to the floor staff and inform them about her decision. His conversations made room for members of her medical team to withdraw from her care if they were unable to support her wishes. One of the residents did have some difficulty, but he told me later that his talk with Stuart enabled him to work through some of his feelings and thereby remain connected with this case. This resident was on his first rotation following medical school, and I can only imagine the dilemma he must have felt. Doctors are trained to save lives.

Mom said most of her good-byes that day. Although everyone around her was sad, we were all aware that death would come as a friend to her. I had been spending nights at the hospital and happened to be awake at 4 A.M. when Mom informed me that she had changed her mind about wanting to die. I sat in total confusion until the hour was civilized enough to call Stuart for some guidance. He wisely counseled me to ask Mom if she remembered what she had said in the middle of the night. She did. She said that she was feeling better and so she no longer wanted to die.

Calls went out to Dr. Ault to rewrite the order for her steroids. Mom finally received them in the early afternoon. But she was clearly confused about medications that day and needed to be told many times what each drug was and what it was for. That was unusual for her. Mom prided herself on her ability to recognize all of her medications and their purpose.

Dr. Ault seemed visibly annoyed at the turn of events and wanted to release Mom from the hospital as soon as possible. She was heavily drugged, communicating rarely although usually clearly, and still concerned about not having the strength to walk to the bathroom. My sister and I had no idea how Mom would be cared for. I knew only that there'd be no discussion of nursing homes. I decided to put off talking about the subject with Mom until after I returned from the ethics committee meeting.

The Society for the Right to Die had offered to send a lawyer to the meeting for my mother, and I mentioned the offer to Stuart a few days earlier. He suggested that the committee members were not there to play an adversarial role and that I could most likely count on their support.

Wise counsel. There was great value in the meeting for me. I learned early in the discussion that they and I were not on opposite sides. Their questions were gentle and pertinent, each aimed at clarifying my mother's wishes.

Stuart was present as an advocate for Mom and did not chair this meeting. His presence was a reminder to me that I was not alone in wanting to support my mother's right to self-determination.

The meeting ended for me on two very positive notes. First, I was told that the committee saw no problem with my mother returning to the hospital if she once again changed her mind about ending treatment. And, second, when I acknowledged my understanding that hospitals were in business to save lives, the chairperson of the committee responded quickly with "Hospitals are also responsible for providing good deaths."

When I returned to Mom's room and shared the gist of the meeting with her, she quietly and firmly informed me that she hadn't changed her mind; she still wanted to die. It took a bit of time to discover that her fear in stopping medication was the fear of not receiving the pain medication. In her confusion, she could no longer trust herself to know what she was taking. I promised to personally give her the Dilaudid and methadone.

July 8, the next day, I followed another of Stuart's wise suggestions and offered Mom her steroids on three separate occasions. Each time, she refused. I never offered them again. One of Dr. Ault's partners, Dr. Klein, was covering for him for a few days and took over Mom's care until she died. Mary Ellen was a gift to us—patient, instructive, caring, unafraid to address the issue at hand. She constantly reassured Mom that there'd be as little pain as possible.

On Saturday, July 9, according to instructions in her Living Will, we switched Mom from oral to intravenous pain medication. Although the house doctors were reluctant to increase dosages when Mom was in obvious pain, they ultimately got it controlled. For much of the time, I still felt that it was us against them and that I needed to protect my mother from potential harm (which translated into not enough painkillers).

When Stuart visited that day, he described some possible scenarios that might take place for Mom prior to her death. The ideal death, he suggested, would be the simultaneous breakdown of all of her functions so that she would just stop breathing.

On July 11, my mother just stopped breathing.

I didn't think I would react to my mother's death as strongly as I have. I expected that nothing would be more painful than her final nineteen months. I was wrong. Anticipatory grief did not relieve me of heavy participation in mourning. For six months, I checked out of life— didn't go to work, stayed in bed reading when I wasn't crying or sleeping, socialized rarely. I became a lay expert on death, dying, and grieving. Through all that's gone on, my husband's love and support have kept me grounded whenever I thought that my world was falling apart.

I am disappointed in myself for not insisting that my mother have a technically proficient specialist who was also a healer, someone capable of seeing beyond a disease, someone gifted in the realm of chronic illness.

I am outraged that no physician took responsibility for addressing and treating my mother's pain until shortly before she died.

I am saddened that my mother's strong need for independence made it difficult to intervene earlier; perhaps I could have helped prevent some of her suffering.

I am baffled by the incredible expertise in our medical system and the incredible inability to coordinate that expertise in a way that supports the people it serves.

I am convinced of the necessity for professional patient advocates. Not every patient has a relative or a Stuart Youngner to protect his or her interests.

I am committed to doctor–patient relationships that are based on collaboration and negotiation. Perhaps medical schools will someday find it appropriate to consider psychological skills as necessary as technical competence.

I am encouraged by the honesty, skill, and compassion that was present in almost every nurse who attended my mother.

I am pleased to have had access to an ethics committee. I wonder, however, if I would have learned of its availability to us had Dr. Stuart Youngner not been involved.

I am indebted to Dr. Stuart Youngner, whose willingness to be a partner through this journey made a significant difference in at least two lives.

I am constantly reminded that there is a time to live and a time to die.

I am honored to be my mother's daughter.

Several of the preceding cases have involved disagreements be-
tween doctors and family members about whether a patient
should be allowed to die. Sometimes the family has wanted to
withdraw life support, but the doctor has been unwilling, and
sometimes the reverse. The locus of disagreement in this case is
different. The patient's family, by choice, played almost no role in
the case, but a strong disagreement arose among staff members
about whether an infant's life support should be withdrawn.

How a Disagreement
over Partiality Helped
Form an Ethics Committee

Loretta M. Kopelman, Ph.D.

PARTIALITY is praised or blamed depending on what we owe to others. An impassioned disagreement arose in a hospital among doctors, nurses, and administrators about how much partiality should be permitted in the long-term care of a chronically and seriously ill infant. Those providing care for this little boy became his advocates, and many of these supporters were also very fond of him. They were criticized, however, for becoming too partial to this child when they allocated goods and services and when they evaluated his prognosis and needs. In what follows, I will describe the conflict about this boy's care, the way it was resolved, and how it helped to form an ethics committee. This disagreement was a sincere moral dispute about how

Loretta Kopelman is Professor and Chair of the Department of Medical Human-
ities, East Carolina University School of Medicine, Greenville, North Carolina. The
author thanks Charles Culver, M.D., Ph.D., and Thomas Irons, M.D., for their many
helpful comments in reviewing this manuscript.

to rank crucial values and understand important duties. I use the description of this debate to illustrate how moral or practical reasoning may be used in consultations.

The Duke

The Duke was born at a nearby hospital in the late 1970s, transferred during a blizzard, and virtually raised at the receiving tertiary-care hospital. Fetal movement had stopped during his mother's eighth month of pregnancy. The Duke was born functionally quadriplegic, essentially unable to move his body from the neck down. The etiology was unknown.

The day after he arrived at the tertiary-care hospital, the director of the neonatal intensive care unit (NICU) called a meeting. There was no formal hospital ethics committee at the time, but a group of us (similar to the committee that later formed) sometimes met to talk over problems. The physicians and nurses were uncertain how to advise the family about what would be the best treatment for their baby. Even with the advantage of hindsight, some are still unsure about this. It seemed very likely this child would not live long even with aggressive care. Most likely, he would always be dependent on a ventilator to breathe. Interventions necessary to sustain his life would be uncomfortable and would often have complications that needed to be balanced against possible benefits to the patient. Given his bleak prognosis, the first reaction of the group was that it would be best for the child not to be treated aggressively but only to be kept comfortable. Enough uncertainty existed about his condition and prognosis, however, that upon reflection we did not recommend this. It was agreed that he needed to be fully supported and evaluated. Our decision to seek a full evaluation seemed appropriate because it allowed us to gather more information. It is important to seek additional relevant information in making a moral decision, although it can be an excuse for avoiding decisions. This was the first of many meetings about The Duke.

At each of our subsequent meetings about The Duke in the NICU, we questioned whether aggressive or only supportive treatment was best for him. Some continued to feel unsure about what was best, concluding that we needed still more information and further evaluations; in the meantime, maximal treatment was provided. Others were increasingly concerned that the aggressive treatment being provided was futile because of his prognosis and inhumane because of his suffering. They said that palliative care was in the child's best interest and intimated that seeking more evaluations was an excuse to avoid the decision. His family did not offer an opinion about what they thought was best for The Duke.

The Duke's family rarely came to see him. At first we thought this might be because they lived some distance from the hospital and, being poor, had problems finding transportation. The social workers encouraged his family to visit, but it gradually became clear that his family did not want to visit The Duke or to be involved in decisions about his care. The social workers concluded that the family had not become attached to the child. There were several reasons for this: the parents did not expect the child to live; the mother and father, who were in their early twenties, were having both financial and marital problems; they had four other children, and this young mother was unable to cope with all that she was given to do. Because their marital discord was severe, the social workers tried to provide family counseling for them.

The Duke did not have a private physician. The neonatologists rotated their duties as attending physicians for the NICU. Each month one of these neonatologists became, in turn, The Duke's physician. All of the neonatologists, however, along with the social workers and nurses caring for him, met regularly. Hence, there was good continuity of care.

The debate in the NICU about The Duke's care abated because he was transferred to the pediatric intensive care unit (PICU) when he was one month old, following an evaluation at another center that confirmed the bleak prognosis. After The Duke was in the PICU for several weeks, the same debate arose there about whether aggressive or palliative care was in The Duke's best interest. The same decision to continue to provide aggressive care was reluctantly reached. The attendings for the PICU also changed monthly, and for almost a year his primary care physician was whoever served as attending for the PICU. Surprisingly, The Duke survived with aggressive care month after month. No regular team meetings about his care occurred during that period.

The damage to The Duke's central nervous system was evaluated and, as expected, found to be permanent. His lungs were in poor condition, and he often struggled to breathe. He was dependent on the ventilator. Seizures associated with apoxic spells and severe respiratory distress were increasingly common in his first year of life. He was never able to feed well by mouth, and getting adequate calories into him was always a struggle. He required a great deal of nursing care. How arrested his development was and what his potential might be were uncertain. One lung was becoming chronically infected, causing repeated debilitating fevers.

He hardly responded to stimuli. The slight reactions he did make, however, seemed very rewarding to many of the nurses who took care of him. Perhaps, as some said, they began to feel like his parents since his own family had stopped coming to see him altogether. Some of the nurses saw encouraging signs and responses that others did not see. The nurses said it was because they spent more time with him. Many of us never saw him respond to anyone in an intentional way. To me, he frequently looked as if he were suffering.

A pediatric pulmonologist agreed to be The Duke's physician on a permanent basis when The Duke was about ten months old, and he became The Duke's primary advocate.

When The Duke was a year and a half old, at a time major health care programs were losing funding, the administration of the hospital became concerned about The Duke's staggering unpaid bill and his continued use of one of only three PICU beds. A hospital utilization committee judged that The Duke should be transferred to a chronic-care facility.

The Duke's condition at eighteen months was as follows: He was totally paralyzed from his shoulders to his lower abdomen; this included his arms and intercostal muscles. He had some voluntary but spastic movement of his lower extremities. After the newborn period he obtained some normal function of his diaphragm. Attempts to wean him from the ventilator, however, failed. He continued to need ventilatory support, as he had from birth. A tracheostomy was necessary. Beginning at two months of age, he had had increasingly frequent episodes of right-upper-lobe atelectasis (collapse of the lung). This was now a constant finding. His right lung functioned very poorly, and the upper lobe was chronically infected. Intravenous antibiotics were required almost continuously. Without them, he would usually develop a high fever within forty-eight to seventy-two hours. Because of thick secretions from his respiratory tract he had to be suctioned frequently. Removal of the chronically infected right lung was contemplated.

The Duke continued to have seizures, most of which were associated with hypoxic (low in oxygen) spells. Medications suppressed his seizures except during periods of severe respiratory distress. The Duke never sucked, and it was hard to feed him by mouth. Most of his nourishment came to him by way of his nasogastric tubes. There was a controversy about his potential for growth and development. Evaluation of his mental development was complicated by his paralysis and tracheostomy. Most agreed that he was quite retarded, but the usual ways to estimate the degree of retardation were blocked. The Duke's family situation had not improved, and there were reports that his parents were planning to divorce.

When the hospital utilization committee ruled that The Duke should go to a chronic-care facility, two hostile camps began to form. They sharply disagreed about whether The Duke should be transferred. Passions were increased by factual disputes: over whether he could survive if transferred to another facility, over whether he could ever be weaned from the ventilator, and over his prognosis, with and without removal of the chronically infected lung. Heated disagreements also erupted among the experts concerning his developmental level at eighteen months. His caregivers found his development, given what he had been through, to be "most promising." They estimated his growth and development as that of a child of "at least 7–8 months." Some pediatricians who examined him disagreed. One said that his development was that of a child of "3–4 months and that is what it will always be." Given The Duke's poor prognosis and suffering, residents and medical students raised troubling questions about what the long-term commitment is to a patient once high technology care is initiated; they asked how many patients like The Duke a hospital can or should support without compensation.

Many of those who had invested time and effort in caring for The Duke were angry because they saw his transfer as a death sentence. Making no claim to being disinterested, they showed their commitment to this child in their everyday willingness to take special care of him. They regarded the hospital as his home and the staff as his family. Talk about what was strictly owed to him as a state resident, as a patient from outside our county, and as a retarded child seemed outrageous and provoked angry responses about people who "took the broad view," "cared only about the bottom line," and "should not be involved in patient care." Some denied that he really cost the hospital time and money: "Somehow we just fit him into our normal duties." Others insisted that whatever the costs, we owed The Duke whatever is in his best interest. They said, "All medical decisions should be based only on what is best for your patient." Quite obviously, they cared for The Duke as an individual; he was a special little boy to them and not just a patient who was taking up an acute-care bed in a tertiary-care facility and whose bill was unpaid. Their fondness and optimism about his condition was apparent in their remarks: "He is a darling little boy who communicates with his eyes"; "He has his ways of letting me know what he wants"; "He has his favorites—those of us he really likes"; "You need special eyes to see what he wants"; "Given what he has been through, he is doing great! We can't stop now."

His room was decorated with toys, cards, and mobiles. At the center was a small boy struggling to breathe. To me, he looked like a baby who was in a lot of pain. Saddened by his suffering, I felt frustrated that we could not do better.

Two camps were polarizing about what should be done about The Duke. In one camp were the pulmonologist who was coordinating the Duke's treatment and the nurses providing his daily care. In the other camp were the physicians and administrators worrying about paying the bills and the availability of bed space for emergencies. Each camp thought the other was using the wrong estimate of what should be provided to the child. Some nurses were criticized for their partiality and for acting like parents to this little boy. Those nurses, however, argued that it would be terrible if they could or should be indifferent or lacking in sympathy to a child so long under their care. Their partiality, they argued, was understandable and even admirable.

Partiality and the Hippocratic Tradition

The pulmonologist and some of the nurses saw no reason to apologize for their advocacy for or partiality to The Duke. They argued that partiality to *your* patient was a part of their professional duty to do good and prevent harm to *their* patients. They were at least correct in that some versions of this duty of beneficence is found in medical, nursing, social work, and other professional codes. I shall refer to them collectively as the *Hippocratic duty of beneficence* because the Hippocratic Oath offers the best-known and most influential expression of this professional duty of beneficence: "I will apply dietetic measures for the benefit of the sick according to my ability and judgment; I will keep them from harm and injustice."

The duty of beneficence is an important tradition, but it should not be understood as recommending absolute partiality for one's own patients. Suppose, for example, that an organ transplantation program collected organs from a large region, promising to distribute them fairly to all in that area. Despite this promise, however, they give all of the organs to *their* patients. This partiality would clearly be unfair because it violates a clear and justified policy about how to allocate goods and services. Even without such a clear policy, however, it would be grounds to criticize the Hippocratic tradition if it encouraged physicians to look out for their own patients and entirely ignore others who are in need.[1] This is especially true when public money is being used.

The Hippocratic tradition, however, need not be understood as requiring unjust partiality.[2] The duty of beneficence as expressed in the Hippocratic tradition requires one to do the best one can for one's patient, but it does not require unfair partiality. One cannot do one's absolute best even for all of the patients under one's care. For one thing, their needs sometimes conflict, or they have to wait their turn. Some other meaning besides absolute partiality to each patient, therefore, must be given to "doing one's best" for patients. If the duty to do good and prevent harm to one's patients is not an absolute duty, what are its limitations? The dispute about The Duke was in part about how to understand the limitations of the duty of beneficence to do what, all things considered, is best for one's patients. The expression "all things considered" shows that we do not think it is an absolute duty but one of many considerations that need to be weighed.

Both camps appealed to the Hippocratic duty of beneficence. This is understandable because it has two different but important interpretations. One is to consider what is best for an *individual* patient. Another is to consider the needs of patients *collectively.* Both the individual and collective concerns for patients are obviously important. As in the case of The Duke, however, they can conflict. Controversies about the appropriate degree of partiality for patients, therefore, may be a sincere moral dispute among people of goodwill who are concerned with different ways to view the duty of beneficence.

Partiality, although justifiable in some cases, may be unwarranted if it is unrealistic or costly or if it violates the rights of others. Had the staff's special interest in The Duke exceeded what was justifiable given his prognosis? Charges that it had were implicit in the comments heard: "I expect this reaction from family but not professionals; this is like dealing with a bunch of parents." "He is like a doll to them. They have invested their own fantasies in him. What can you do?" "If anyone tries to do anything, be prepared to deal with a lot of unreality from the floor." "I hope someone will deal with the issue of the improper use of technology; he should not have been put on the respirator to begin with." "This is sentiment not reason operating." "How many acutely ill but fully curable children have been turned away because he occupies one of the three PICU beds? It's wrong." "What we could accomplish with that money. He has no future." "The strain on the staff is terrible when a child like that is on the floor. I hope someone will say 'enough suffering, no more.'" "What we need is a willingness to cooperate with the chronic care facilities, not to simply assume they cannot handle things." "They think if it feels right it is right."

Critics claimed that those caring for The Duke had allowed their fondness for him to capture too much of the institution's resources and to color their assessments of The Duke's condition, prognosis, and suffering. Despite such charges of partiality and a lack of professionalism, The Duke's physician (the pulmonologist) and nurses caring for The Duke held firm. Believing they had a duty to protect their patient, who they felt would die if transferred to a chronic-care facility, they resisted pressure to discharge The Duke.

The confrontation between the two camps threatened to blow up beyond the walls of the hospital. Despite objections, a date was set for his transfer. Some said that if he was transferred, they would "go to the newspapers," "get a lawyer," or "take it to the courts." To try to defuse the situation, the pulmonologist who was directing The Duke's care planned a grand rounds. He hoped that we could use the grand rounds to review The Duke's history and physical findings, as well as the issues. After the grand rounds he planned to have those most involved move to a conference setting for further discussion. He would speak at the grand rounds, and he asked me to be the other speaker. He asked me to be the sole speaker if he was too upset that day. He spoke and was fine.

My contribution at the grand rounds was to try to clarify the issues and to structure the discussion. One of the things I tried to show, as discussed above, was that there were different ways to understand the Hippocratic duty of beneficence. I tried to show that both disputing camps could honestly claim that they were trying to do good and prevent harm to patients because the Hippocratic duty of beneficence has two different interpretations (individual and collective) that can lead to conflicts about what ought to be done. The Hippocratic tradition in itself offers no guidance about what degree of partiality is unacceptable in specific cases. Thus, it cannot solve these disputes. Both camps might appeal to the Hippocratic tradition but could not use it to settle the problem of what to do when there was a conflict about how to distribute goods and services fairly. Estimates about what degree of partiality is justifiable in such cases is a complicated moral and social issue.

Partiality and Justice

The debate over The Duke's care had become polarized because people were using different estimates of what was justly owed to patients under their care. In what follows I will argue, as I did in the grand rounds, that this is an example of a controversy about how to allocate goods and services justly in a society. How should we fairly allocate our health care services? Insofar as we want a health care system that promotes empathic care, some partiality may have to be tolerated even when state funds are used. The degree of partiality is not a matter of what we feel to be right, however, but a moral decision with a social dimension about how we would all want to be treated in similar circumstances. In a just system there is a proper consideration for all persons, but consideration for all must begin with concern for particular individuals. When we care about particular individuals, however, it is inevitable that we will feel partial to them. Thus, in a just society we encourage people to care about each other as individuals, accepting that this will foster some partiality. And if we want people to be cared for as individuals in the health care system, we should not be surprised that partiality results.

Philosophers Aristotle, David Hume, and Simone Weil have argued that spontaneous affection for individuals is a necessary part of a just system. Hume called acts by which we respond to others out of compassion or friendship, without any thought of impartial schemes, "the virtues of the heart."[3] It is important to promote the virtues of the heart, such as compassion, because they foster fellow feeling, empathy, and mutual concern. Such a response, he wrote, focuses on the needs of others, moving us without thoughts of schemes, systems, or consequences. "A parent flies to the relief of his child; transported by that natural sympathy which actuates him, and which affords no leisure to reflect on the sentiments or conduct of the rest of mankind in like circumstances. A generous man cheerfully embraces an opportunity of serving his friend."[3] Aristotle also pointed out that the demands or acts of friendship may be unique and, like Hume, argued that friendships have utility in fostering mutual concern in a just state.[4] Simone Weil also thought our concern for justice and well-being for people in general was borne out in a concern for individuals.[5] Aristotle, Hume, and Weil argued that such spontaneous concern must be encouraged in a just society. Such spontaneous affection will cause partiality. A purely impartial system may be less acceptable to us all than a system that tolerates some degree of partiality.

To understand the weakness of either a purely partial or a purely impartial system, it is helpful to distinguish between the *ethics of friendship,* where we think a high degree of partiality is justifiable, and the *ethics of impartial justice,* where we think it is not.[2] One strength of relying on compassion or friendship to direct action is that it encourages our concern for each other, not as representatives of some group but as individuals. This moves us away from minimalistic positions about what we strictly owe each other and, if it does not infringe on the rights of others, promotes goodwill and fellow feeling between people. It encourages us to be more generous, caring, and merciful.

Feelings of compassion alone are dangerous guides for conduct, however. First, trusting our feelings of compassion can mislead us about what is really best. A persistent criticism of those who advocated maximal care for The Duke, for example, was that they did not "see" his high level of suffering. Thus, what appeared to his advocates in their enthusiasm to be compassionate, critics said, on reflection was not. They were trusting their feelings without being critical.

Another potential problem with reliance on feelings of compassion alone is that it is not fair to have a general policy where distribution of goods and services depend on favoritism. The needs and rights of others may be unjustly overlooked or set aside in our feelings, enthusiasm, or sentimentality for a preferred few.

In setting policies, resolving conflicts, and balancing needs, wants, and resources fairly, impartial schemes may be complex. This complexity may appear to show a lack of sympathy to the plight of particular individuals; it may appear to show a meanness of spirit and seem to thwart emotions that make us feel good about what we do. In some cases, however, as in certain of the transplant programs, standards of fairness, eligibility, and impartiality can offer more altruism and protection for us all than the heartfelt, spontaneous sentimentality that favors those before us. By ignoring fairness for feelings, the entire procurement and distribution system may be threatened.

Those trying to apply general and more impartial rules to this little boy were criticized as uncaring. The interests of society to limit costs, however, may be at odds with interests of particular patients and their families. Administrators and committees may be increasingly called on to represent a disinterested view about what can be provided to patients, based on impartial considerations such as cost and prognosis. This is an issue of how we as a society are prepared to distribute goods and services given our finite resources.

We adopt impartial schemes because we see it is fair and useful to do so. The goal of such an impartial system is to determine what each of us would want under conditions of equality, or when we do not know where we would find ourselves. None of us knows whether or not he or she will be the person getting partial treatment when important resources are limited, so we prefer an impartial scheme. It is fair and useful to make a plan about how to treat all similarly in similar circumstances. The system is an impartial, fair way to solve conflicts or disagreements about how to allocate scarce goods or services in a way generally acceptable to informed people of goodwill.

Many of the parties in the dispute about The Duke seemed to think that it was very clear what degree of partiality is defensible for patients like The Duke. But it was not clear to me, and it still is not. Moreover, justifying what degree of partiality is just requires us to look at the needs and resources of a particular society. If money is to be left for schooling, roads, mass transit, and museums, then some limitations must be set on health care spending. If public money is used, then we need to indicate how much of our health care dollars should be spent for certain conditions. It would be imprudent, for example, to spend all of our money for terminal care and none for preventive care. Within some specific framework, we as a society can determine when it is just to allow some partiality for the sake of fostering an empathic health care system.

Those taking care of The Duke thought partiality was defensible because of their professional duties to provide him with the best medical care possible. They argued that the system could afford it and that partiality was the direct result of the empathic care that they had been encouraged to give. Some degree of partiality may be acceptable in a just health care system that seeks empathic care as well as some degree of impartiality in the distribution of goods and services.

The Outcome

After many more discussions, it was decided that The Duke would not be transferred to the chronic-care facility and that his chronically infected lung would be removed. To the amazement of many, The Duke was then weaned from the ventilator for up to a day a time; however, the ventilator never left his room. Because his family had been unable to cope with him a foster family was found. He improved enough to leave the hospital for the first time in his life at twenty months of age.

At his good-bye party the attachment of some of the nurses to this baby was made clear by the large hand-painted signs that decorated the walls: "We love you"; "I will miss you too"; "You will always know us"; and "You are family."

There was a moving story in the Sunday paper, complete with many pictures, entitled "The Duke Goes Home." Presented as a success story of modern medicine, it never mentioned his life of pain, the controversies, the cost to the county for a nonresident, or the need for better support facilities for disabled children. Cynics said that sort of reality does not sell newspapers.

He was back in the hospital a week and a half later. For the next year, he was out of the hospital only briefly. Finally, it became clear to everyone that treatment was inhumane and futile. A memo was sent to all who had been involved with his care. It said that his families (foster and biological) and physicians agreed that The Duke's continuing central nervous system deterioration and the progressive pulmonary disease made aggressive treatment by mechanical ventilation inappropriate. Comfort care, antibiotics, and other supports would be given. The memo said that the families were free to change their decision. They did not. Everyone agreed about what to do and why they ought to do it. The consensus was genuine. They came to agree that treatment was inhumane and futile.

Using Moral Reasoning in Consultations

No agreement was ever reached about what ought to be fairly allocated to patients such as The Duke. Agreement was elusive because different positions seemed morally justified. This was unusual because most of the time agreement is reached in ethics consultations. Moral solutions to problems require a certain sort of defense, and in the course of using this method of practical reasoning we usually come to agree.

In this section I want to clarify what this method of moral or practical reasoning is and indicate a series of questions that might be useful to keep in mind when conducting consultations. This method can help us resolve disputes or locate the nature of our disagreements.

To put forth one's opinion *as moral*, one must be willing to justify it in a certain way.[6] That is, one must be willing to seek clarity in stating the problem and all relevant information, to defend choices with reasons, and to reconsider views in light of new data. Seeking a moral defense of one's position also requires that one not be egotistical but rather be willing to apply the reasons to all, universally and impartially, even to oneself (the Golden Rule expresses this). One must seek to assess one's reasons critically in relation to other relevant considerations, such as legal, social, or religious traditions, or other stable views about how we should act or what we should be. It also requires a willingness to be sensitive to moral conflicts or problems, to beliefs about what is compassionate, and to the feelings, preferences, or rights of others. Like the scientific method, this kind of moral reasoning is a goal we seek, and none of us should claim with certainty that it has been reached. For example, as in the debate over The Duke, we cannot be certain we have all of the relevant data or that the "factual" assessments are uncolored by what we expect or want to find.

This method of moral or practical reasoning may be used in consultations by centering it around the following questions:

1. What is the problem?

2. Are there other or better ways to view it?

3. What data are relevant? Are you using the best information? How good are your data?

4. What are the options?

5. What are the likely consequences of the different options?

6. What rights, duties, or values are important? If there is a conflict, what is the weightiest consideration?

7. What are the weaknesses of your view?

8. How would you want to be treated in these circumstances?

Consider these questions as they apply to The Duke. Part of what caused the angry, heartfelt disputes about The Duke was that for a long time there was little agreement about what data were relevant or reliable, what the consequences were likely to be, or even how to state the problem.

Over time the hard lines between the two camps about how to frame the problem softened, and sympathy for other ways to view the problem emerged (see questions 1 and 2). Some doctors and nurses who took care of The Duke initially saw the problem as: What can we do that is best for this baby? They understood "the best" to mean whatever would prolong his life. Others thought that what was best for him, given his condition, was palliative care. Still others thought that it was necessary to consider the needs of children in the region, given our limited resources. Many of us saw the controversy about The Duke as stemming from our society's unwillingness to confront allocation issues in health care or to address the needs of chronically ill persons.

Questions about what data were relevant and whether we had the best possible information (see question 3) were always difficult because The Duke's condition made it hard to gather the relevant data and because the experts disagreed about his condition and prognosis. The consensus about The Duke's care resulted only from his eventual deterioration. Factual disagreements and uncertainties also affected the decisions about what options were open to deal with the situation. At one extreme, some refused to think of anything but the tertiary-care facility as an option for The Duke's care; others saw that only a chronic-care facility was appropriate. On reflection, both of these options were rejected in favor of one advocated by the social workers and one of the ambulatory pediatricians. They argued that home care was a realistic goal. The decision that prevailed was to continue aggressive care, to try to wean him from the ventilator, and to seek eventual foster care placement (see questions 4 and 5). For some it seemed a wonderful choice, for others the "least worst" given the situation. As it turned out, home care was a realistic goal because The Duke's foster family was exceptionally good (some said saintly).

In clarifying the problems, data, and options, it became easier to acknowledge and agree on what general values were at stake (see question 6). It was not the "do-gooders" against the "bottom-liners" as each of the camps was at first inclined to call the other. Rather, over time, we were able to see the weaknesses of either a purely partial or a purely impartial system of health care (see question 7). It became clear that whatever degree of partiality is acceptable, it must be available to all.

In answering the question about how you would want to be treated in these circumstances (question 8), you should consider that you might be any one of the parties involved, including the person who cannot get a PICU bed. Although you might want to know your situation, justice requires that everyone's interests be considered equally. The physicians, nurses, and families of sick children in an outlying hospital want to find ICU beds in the nearest tertiary-care hospital; no doubt they would be unhappy to find admissions closed because a child who could have been transferred was not. In contrast, if you were taking care of The Duke or were a member of his family, you might want what is best for him; if you believe he might do better to stay, you would want this treatment. As we have seen, two different focuses of the Hippocratic duty of beneficence (individual and collective) can result in different decisions about how one should act. But in moral or practical reasoning one tries to envision disinterested or impartial views of what ought to be done. To test when partiality is fair or defensible, imagine that you do not know whether you are the patient, the family, an advocate for the person in the facility, or an advocate for the person seeking admission to it. A just society should clarify the degree of partiality that is acceptable in social programs. Arguably, we lack a well-defined policy, so it is not surprising that such disagreements erupt when money is tight.

The Duke's Legacy: Agreement Is Not Everything

It is hard to say how much The Duke suffered through his short life, but one of his legacies was the formation of a hospital ethics committee. In discussing The Duke, it became clear that it would be useful to have such a committee. One goal of an ethics committee is to help resolve conflicts about the care of patients. Since there was so much controversy about The Duke, it might seem that forming an ethics committee to resolve disputes is an odd legacy for The Duke to leave us. But although agreement is one important goal of an ethics committee, it should not be thought of as the *primary* goal. Agreement can be reached by immoral means such as by stifling discussions or merely authorizing what some powerful person wants. An ethics committee can serve as an arm of risk management for the institution, use secondhand data, promote "group-think," or serve as a "rubber-stamp committee."[7] Such consultations discourage the critical assessment of the relevant data, values, duties, rights, or principles.[8] Although committees can be used to thwart the ideals of the practical moral judgment, they can also foster these goals. Ideally, ethics committee consultations promote thoughtful, open, and informed discussions about what ought to be done. In addition to promoting sensitivity to the general as well as the unique features of situations, they can help educate, develop policies, check prognoses, and offer support. The ethics committee was a good legacy for The Duke to leave us.

Notes

1. R. Veatch, *A Theory of Medical Ethics* (New York: Basic Books, 1981).

2. Loretta Kopelman, "Justice and the Hippocratic Tradition of Acting for the Good of the Sick," in *Ethics and Critical Care Medicine* ed. John C. Moskop and Loretta M. Kopelman (Dordrecht, Holland: D. Reidel Publishing Company, 1985), 79–104. Portions of this paper were used directly or adapted for use herein.

3. David Hume, *An Inquiry Concerning the Principles of Morals,* (LaSalle, Ill.: Open Court Publishing Company, 1953), 156 (original work published 1751). References in the text are to the 1953 edition, reprinted from the 1777 edition.

4. Aristotle, *Nicomachean Ethics.*

5. Simone Weil, *First and Last Notebooks*, trans. R. Rees (London: University Press, 1970).

6. W. Frankena, *Ethics* (2nd ed.) (Englewood Cliffs, N.J.: Prentice-Hall, 1973).

7. B. Lo, "Behind Closed Doors: Promises and Pitfalls of Ethics Committees," *New England Journal of Medicine* 317 (July 2, 1987): 46–49.

8. S. Perry, "The NIH Consensus Development Program: A Decade Later," *New England Journal of Medicine* 317 (August 20, 1987): 485–88.

This is the first of two cases that do not have as their central moral dilemma whether a patient should be allowed to die. In each of these two cases there was a division among staff members about whether to accede to or overrule the wishes of a patient who wanted to be discharged to his own home rather than to a nursing home.

Rationality and Competence in Hospital Discharge Planning: The Case of Mr. Cary

William A. Nelson, Ph.D.

Andrew S. Pomerantz, M.D.

DURING the first week of January the chair of the Ethics Advisory Committee (W.N.) received a call from Susan, the coordinator of the inpatient rehabilitation unit. It concerned an ethical problem about the placement of one of their patients. Mr. Cary wanted to be discharged to his home, but the staff felt that his physical needs were too great to allow a home placement. The problem was not considered an emergency, so a meeting was scheduled for the next day with Susan to talk about the case. A nurse member of the Ethics Advisory Committee (EAC) and the chairperson met with Susan.

William Nelson is Associate Professor of Clinical Psychiatry at Dartmouth Medical School, Hanover, New Hampshire, and Chief of the Chaplain Service, Veterans Administration Medical Center, White River Junction, Vermont. Andrew Pomerantz is Assistant Professor of Clinical Psychiatry at Dartmouth Medical School and Director of the Psychiatry Consultation–Liaison Service, Veterans Administration Medical Center. The opinions expressed here are the authors' and do not necessarily represent the views of the Veterans Administration.

143

The thirty-eight-bed rehabilitation unit is an autonomously functioning ward located within the acute-care hospital. It is directed by a nurse coordinator. Day-to-day medical care is provided by nurses, various therapists, a physician's assistant who is backed up by physicians, and other health care providers. The staff physicians are called on for acute medical problems, but ordinary patient management is directed by the rehabilitation staff. Patients needing rehabilitation prior to discharge often come to the unit from the acute-care setting.

In meeting with a clinician who seeks advice from the EAC, we try to determine two factors as clearly and accurately as we can: What are the facts of the case and what is the moral dilemma? Many "ethical dilemmas" turn out to be disagreements over facts. These disagreements can occur among the staff as well as between the patient and the staff. If agreement on the facts of the case can be achieved, moral dilemmas often disappear. It is important for ethics consultants to develop skill in ferreting out a case's factual basis. Terms like "hopeless" or "aggressive measures" or "heroic treatment" cannot be accepted without determining what such terms mean in a particular case.

The Case

Mr. Cary was a previously healthy fifty-year-old junior high school social studies teacher who had been in a car accident in the summer of 1977. He transected his spinal cord just below the neck, and after a year in a spinal cord injury rehabilitation center, he remained paraplegic (paralyzed from the chest down). Over the next three years, he suffered from chronic pain, unrelieved by multiple surgical procedures on his spinal cord and brain, but he continued to function well at work in a wheelchair. In 1981 he was named teacher of the year in his school district. By early 1982, however, his wife had left him and he was in danger of losing his job; in the fall he took a nonlethal overdose of narcotic analgesics. At that time he suffered from severe chronic pain and had minimum exercise tolerance because of breathing problems, and his medical problem list now contained thirteen diagnoses. He stated that whether or not to go on living was a "daily decision."

During a hospital admission in 1983, the staff, concerned about his ability to manage at home, encouraged him to move to a more controlled environment. However, he returned home and continued there except for occasional brief hospitalizations until he broke his leg in a fall in April 1987. At that time he was admitted to the hospital for orthopedic treatment. Following the acute phase of his treatment he was transferred to the rehabilitation unit, where he remained for nearly a year. Mr. Cary thought the purpose of the admission was for rehabilitation so that he could return home. The staff, however, believed he was too functionally impaired to live alone and felt discharge should be to a supervised setting. This difference in opinion was never openly acknowledged because the staff believed that eventually Mr. Cary would realize that he could no longer live alone.

Over the course of hospitalization, Mr. Cary declined physically and lost his endurance for the vigorous physical therapy necessary to regain sufficient function to return home. Despite intensive pharmacological and behavioral treatment, his pain persisted, self-rated at an average of 7.5 to 8.0 on a 0–10 scale. He never regained the ability to move himself to and from his wheelchair, and the staff recommended placement in a nursing home. Mr. Cary steadfastly declined nursing home placement and insisted he would prefer to go home and "give it a try." He stated repeatedly that he would rather die than live in a nursing home.

Psychiatric involvement with Mr. Cary during his current admission began on July 1, about three months after admission. At that point he was frequently expressing suicidal thoughts. He was being treated with antidepressants and substantial doses of narcotic analgesics to diminish pain. During visits with the psychiatry team (a staff psychiatrist, a second-year psychiatry resident, and a third-year medical student) he frequently talked about his helplessness and his dependency on others, who, in his perception, always seemed to let him down. Mr. Cary denied that his own behavior ever contributed to these conflicts. He was in a great deal of pain, which increased his isolation. He seldom saw his family: he had no contact with his ex-wife, a son who lived in a nearby town came to visit occasionally, and his daughters were living out of state. While he was hospitalized, his home was robbed, a fact he discovered during a four-hour pass. He lost several thousand dollars worth of stereo and woodworking equipment in the burglary, which left him feeling even more powerless than before. This unfortunate occurrence increased his desire to go home and regain a sense of control over his life.

Conversations with Mr. Cary usually focused on nonpsychological matters. He enjoyed talking about science, something that always made him feel better. He took particular delight in teaching his doctors something new. Whenever the discussion turned to closely held thoughts and feelings, however, he always made it clear that his most cherished possession besides his intellect was his sense of independence. If he couldn't have that, he said, the price he would pay in pain each day in an institution simply was too great.

The goal of Mr. Cary's hospitalization was to regain the strength he had lost during the prolonged immobilization required for his leg to heal. Throughout the hospitalization, however, his involvement in physical and occupational therapy was erratic, and during the fall and early winter it became clear to the staff that he had not regained the strength necessary to live alone successfully. Since his admission he had lost the ability to move to and from his wheelchair, and after a thorough evaluation, the staff believed it would be impossible for him to regain that necessary skill. During a meeting with the rehabilitation staff and with his son, Mr. Cary was informed that the staff could only recommend permanent placement in a long-term nursing home. When he balked, he was informed that any other disposition plan would be tantamount to "setting himself up to fail" and would be unacceptable.

Mr. Cary asked to think over the options for several days. He explored the possibility of having a track set up in the ceiling of his home, using winches and other tools to allow him to move in and out of his wheelchair and to move himself around. He continued to complain about his pain and reminded his caretakers that it often made life unbearable for him. At one time he remarked, "Why does everyone make such a big deal about just staying alive? What's so great about being in pain all the time?" He asked many questions about the available nursing home and said his greatest fear was that he would be "surrounded" with patients who had Alzheimer's disease and would have nobody to talk to. Although he understood that the odds were not in his favor, Mr. Cary chose to decline medical advice and instead to return home, stating, "It is something I have to do." He said that if he failed at home, he would try a nursing home; and if that failed, suicide would be another alternative. The staff, fearing that physical decline at home could be very rapid and lead to his death, felt that they would be colluding with a suicide plan if they were to discharge him home. In good conscience they could not accept his decision and asked for a formal psychiatric evaluation of his competency. The nurse coordinator of the unit asked that he be evaluated for an involuntary commitment to the state mental hospital because she felt that his desire to go home was in truth a suicide plan. From the staff's perspective, Mr. Cary's need for independence was far less important than his life. They believed it was either irrational or suicidal for an individual to "Live Free or Die" (the state motto on Mr. Cary's license plate).

The psychiatry team viewed the request as a measure of how desperate the staff members were feeling. They felt they had done their best to mobilize the patient and return him to a more functional status, but he had physically declined instead. Now he was choosing against their advice and picking a course that could result in his death. Mr. Cary had a certain facility for leaving others feeling as though they had not done enough for him, and the staff was no exception. They felt that if he went home and died, it would be their "fault." The staff felt a paternalistic decision was warranted and were looking for grounds for overriding Mr. Cary's wishes.

Although a legal declaration of competency can be made only by a court, psychiatrists are often called on when the need for a patient care decision is urgent or as a prelude to engaging the legal system when time is not critical. Usually, the evaluation assesses a specific area of functioning because incompetency is not necessarily a global phenomenon. One can suffer from dementia and still be competent in some areas and capable of making certain kinds of decisions. The most frequent request concerns competency to refuse medication or other treatment. To be competent, a patient must understand that he or she is being asked to make a decision and that the decision will determine the medical treatment. Usually, the examiner will try to elicit the patient's understanding of his or her overall situation, the treatment(s) offered, the risks and benefits of the treatment, and the consequences of declining treatment (or picking one treatment in preference to another). It is critical that the questions be formulated in a manner that elicits spontaneous statements of the patient's understanding. A general principle in interviewing is that the more direct the question, the less reliable the response; for example, "Did the doctor tell you you might die without the medicine?" compared to "What did the doctor tell you might happen without the medicine?"

Psychiatrists are often asked to make competency evaluations when patients refuse a medication or a treatment. Evaluating a patient's competence to decide where he should be discharged occurs less often, but in recent years with increasing frequency. As hospitals are required to be cost-efficient, there is pressure for faster discharges. To clarify the questions in Mr. Cary's case, the discharge plan was viewed as a proposed treatment and his refusal to comply as a refusal of treatment.

The evaluation of competency was straightforward in Mr. Cary's case. Simply stated, he was able to state the essential facts of his case: that the staff was recommending a specific treatment (nursing home placement) with the anticipated benefit of keeping him alive in a supportive environment and that his choice to act against that recommendation ran a risk of leading directly to his death. He understood and could state the specifics of the staff's concerns, and he even quoted their estimate that his odds of surviving at home were roughly one in five. Mr. Cary felt death would be better than a life of continued suffering in an institution. He was willing to take the risk of dying at home. He also expressed doubt that his decline at home would be precipitous enough to prevent his return to the hospital. Because he understood and appreciated the relevant information, the psychiatry consult team viewed him as competent to give a valid consent or in this case a valid refusal of the proposed placement.

Although he seemed competent to make the decision, the underlying question on the mind of the staff was "This decision doesn't make any sense; do we have to honor it?" Although a few psychiatrists consider rationality a part of competency,[1,2] we prefer to distinguish between the two. Competency refers to the ability to make an informed decision (i.e., the "process" of decision making), and rationality refers to the quality of that decision once it has been made (i.e., the "result" of the decision-making process). A rational decision is one for which the patient can cite "adequate reasons."[3]

The staff hoped that if Mr. Cary's decision could be deemed irrational, then it could be overridden. In his talks with the psychiatry team he repeatedly stated that he thought death was "overrated," that chronic pain was "underrated" and that no one could fully understand what life was like for him, constantly in pain and unable even to move himself into a less uncomfortable position. In his view the only thing that would make life tolerable after discharge would be to return to his own home, where he could resume his hobbies, including woodworking and birdwatching. If he had to give up his remaining shreds of independence, in addition to the pain he suffered every day (despite having had neurosurgical, pharmacological, electronic, and behavioral treatments for pain), life would not be worth living. This explanation supplied an adequate reason for the risk he was taking. Thus, there were no grounds on which to act paternalistically and override his decision.

Despite detailed explanations of the reasoning used by the consulting psychiatrist, the staff could not accept any decision that might lead to Mr. Cary's death. They simply postponed making any discharge plans. The psychiatry consult team fielded increasingly agitated complaints from staff members who said they could not abide by Mr. Cary's decision because it would certainly lead to his death. A consultation with the EAC was therefore set up by the unit staff; this was welcomed by the psychiatry team. The staff psychiatrist (A.P.) dealt with the conflict of also being on the ethics committee by speaking only as Mr. Cary's psychiatrist.

Mr. Cary and the EAC

Discharge planning is a common practice in hospitals and is not usually perceived as ethically problematic. However, in recent years issues of cost containment, quality assurance, and patient involvement in discharge planning have taken on increased significance. One level of decision making concerns the determination of the appropriate placement options. Another significant issue is determining who should make the final placement decision. Does the ultimate decision-making responsibility lie with the patient, the family, the institution, or society as a whole?[4-6]

The EAC carefully reviewed the facts of the case and came to the same conclusion as had the psychiatry team: Mr. Cary was competent, and his decision to return home, while risky, was not irrational. The committee did not believe that forcing institutional placement on Mr. Cary would be morally justified; neither did they believe that postponing his discharge home was warranted.

The attorney member of the committee was contacted concerning the legal ramifications of the case. This is not an uncommon committee practice. The law does not determine what the EAC will advise, but it is important to know if there are applicable legal rulings and if the committee's morally based advice exposes the care providers, the hospital, or even the committee to risk. Our attorney's opinion was that the courts would almost certainly support the advice given.

On occasion the EAC may give ethical advice that does marginally increase the hospital's legal risk, such as informing a patient about medical errors that have occurred in his care. The EAC should be aware of the legal ramifications of any recommended course of action and of what might be done to minimize hospital liability. This information should be communicated to the person requesting the ethics consultation. The EAC's attorney suggested that a meeting be held, if Mr. Cary agreed, with as many of his family members as possible. The meeting would be an opportunity to explore the placement decision with Mr. Cary, the staff, and the family. The family could hear the patient's thinking and his decision. The family would understand that the patient's desire to go home was against the recommendations of the staff. If the placement should result in problems, the family would not then believe that the staff or hospital had pushed the patient into returning home. The substance of the meeting would be documented in Mr. Cary's chart.

A family meeting was called; however, Mr. Cary's son was the only family member able to attend. During the meeting, problems with home placement were reviewed. The son agreed with the staff that home placement would be risky, and he pleaded with his father to reconsider his decision. Mr. Cary said he would think about the discussion, but within days he indicated that he was adamant about going home. Again, the staff was disappointed in his decision.

Following the ethics committee review, arrangements for Mr. Cary's discharge proceeded slowly, and over the next month they ground to a halt. Several members of the staff were not satisfied with either the EAC or the psychiatric consultations, and some were openly angry. This was not an easy time for us. It was the first time a consultation had met such opposition. We reviewed our thinking but came to the same conclusion. During this time we often stopped by the rehabilitation unit to talk with the staff about the case, in an attempt to clarify our thinking for them. We wanted to avoid an emotional polarization between the EAC and the unit staff, and we believe we were largely successful.

During Mr. Cary's extended hospitalization the issue of the costs of his care was rarely discussed, probably because he was in a V.A. hospital.

In retrospect, we believe the EAC should have gone to the hospital administration and urged Mr. Cary's discharge. We believed that prolonging his hospitalization was ethically unjustified and also financially costly. The economic issue for the hospital should not dictate health care decision making for an individual patient, but it cannot be completely ignored. Even in the V.A. health system the issues of cost containment are of growing significance and will increasingly be an issue for EACs.

Another competency evaluation was requested by the unit staff and was performed by psychiatry. The staff continued to be upset by what they perceived as the patient's intransigence. The recommendation from psychiatry was to set a discharge date and proceed with the plan. The weight of the EAC opinion enabled psychiatry to add a notation at the bottom of the chart: "I believe this is consistent with the recommendations of the EAC." Being able to do so made the limb the psychiatry staff felt it was standing on seem sturdier.

About two months after the ethics consultation was requested, the decision to discharge Mr. Cary to his home was made. This followed multiple meetings, consultations, and conversations. Many of these discussions focused on the frustration of the rehabilitation staff that this patient in whom they had invested so much might soon die. Over time, however, there came to be general acceptance by the staff of the justifiability of allowing Mr. Cary to return home.

Throughout this time, Mr. Cary remained a passive object of discussion. Whenever asked, he repeated his wish to return home, yet he displayed no overt irritation at the delay in arranging discharge. Instead, he became a more "difficult" patient, increasing his demands on the staff, decreasing his compliance with treatment, and becoming increasingly critical of the care he was receiving.

Outcome

After the decision to discharge Mr. Cary to his home was made and a date set, the team began to make arrangements with outside agencies to provide whatever help was available in his community. Schedules were worked out with visiting nurses from the community and the hospital. Arrangements were initiated to provide "lifeline" telephone service to the hospital through a home-placed call button and to provide for Meals-on-Wheels on a regular basis. When the discharge date arrived, he returned to his home to live for the first time in nearly a year. At the time he left, he spoke little of his own plight but talked at length about sports and how the underdogs often can succeed despite the expectations of others.

Within a month, Mr. Cary called for an ambulance and was returned to the acute-care ward of the hospital. As predicted by some of the staff, he had been unable to manage essential self-care at home, and he arrived with a bowel impaction and mild dehydration. He was chagrined by what he perceived to be his "failure" and said he would accept transfer to a long-term facility on at least a trial basis. A placement was arranged, and he was scheduled for transfer three weeks later. One week prior to this discharge he began to question whether he might really be better off trying it at home again, so psychiatry and the EAC were consulted. The psychiatry team and the EAC felt that his talk of "trying it at home" was reflective of his ongoing ambivalence over his options. Following several conversations he decided to go to the nursing home. The recommendation was to proceed with placement at the scheduled time to the nursing home.

Mr. Cary was transferred to the nursing home without objection on the scheduled discharge date. From the beginning of his stay there, however, he found fault with all aspects of the facility and asked visitors to help him leave and return home. He endured his new environment for two months before arranging with two friends to carry him out of the nursing home unnoticed during the night and return him to his own home.

Once there, Mr. Cary took more active charge of his own fate. Rather than relying on social workers to arrange support services for him, he took the initiative himself and contacted the hospital, his psychiatrist, and local social agencies. Three weeks later, after breathing difficulties prompted a call to the visiting nurse, he died suddenly while sitting in his wheelchair. Autopsy and toxicology studies revealed his death to be secondary to acute respiratory failure with no evidence of suicide.

The EAC reviewed Mr. Cary's case after receiving word of his death. Despite the unfortunate outcome, we felt our advice had been morally appropriate because Mr. Cary's decision to be discharged home was a valid refusal of institutional care and consistent with his values. We continued to be upset by the long delay in his discharge. Our committee, like most, functions in an advisory role, but we felt we should have been more aggressive from the beginning in pushing for home placement. Because of our desire to maintain an advisory role and not appear intrusive, we failed to be the advocate that Mr. Cary needed. If a similar case should be presented to the committee in the future, we would probably play a more assertive role, even if that meant directly confronting the physician director of the rehabilitation unit or going to the administration. In taking such a tack, the EAC could be viewed as mandating decisions and could create an atmosphere of mistrust. This is the only case ever brought to our EAC that has raised this problem for us. Despite the potential negative ramifications from acting in a confrontational manner, EACs may on occasion have an ethical responsibility to do just that.

The psychiatry department also reviewed Mr. Cary's case. Although

the logic behind the assessment of Mr. Cary's competence and rationality appeared sound, we felt we might have been remiss by being too
respectful of the dynamics of the ward itself. Although managed day to
day by the nursing staff, the ward also includes a physician medical
director and a physician assistant who writes orders as the agent for the
medical director. Several other physicians are assigned to cover the
unit. Traditional tensions between doctors and nurses and physician
assistants frequently complicate the environment. Almost from the
outset, Mr. Cary was in frequent conflict with the physician assistant
and commented that he'd never met his attending physician. As a
matter of practice, the physicians who cover the unit recognize that
nursing is in charge of the unit and avoid involvement there. The
physician assistant is then left as the only nonnursing person doing
clinical work on the ward and would have a great deal of difficulty
writing an order that all of his co-workers thought was contraindicated.
Attempts to involve the attending physician were fruitless, but in retrospect the psychiatry staff felt that they should have been more insistent
that he intervene and take the unpopular route of ordering discharge
when Mr. Cary made his choice.

Notes

1. B. Chell, "Competency: What It Is, What It Isn't, and Why It Matters," in
Medical Ethics, ed. J. Monagle and D. Thomasma (Rockville, Mo.: Aspen Publications, 1988) 99–110.

2. P. Appelbaum and T. Grisso, "Assessing Patient's Capacities to Consent to
Treatment," 1988, *New England Journal of Medicine* 319(25) (1988): 1635–8.

3. C. Culver and B. Gert, *Philosophy in Medicine* (New York: Oxford University
Press, 1982), chaps. 2, 3.

4. A. Caplan, D. Callahan, and J. Haas, "Ethical and Policy Issues in Rehabilitation Medicine," *Hastings Center Report* 17(4) (August/September 1987): 1–20.

5. M. Abramson, "Ethical Dilemmas for Social Workers in Discharge Planning,"
Social Work in Health Care 6(4) (Summer 1981): 33–42.

6. M. Abramson, "A Model for Organizing an Ethical Analysis of the Discharge
Planning Process," *Social Work in Health Care* 9(1) (Fall 1983): 45–52.

*The staff disagreement in the preceding case led to a
lengthy, quiet, grim impasse. In Ruth Purtilo's case it
leads to near-pandemonium. Purtilo has chosen to write
about an unsettling case that had an uncertain closure.
Most ethics consultation cases are not like that; but a
few are, and it is fitting that one be included here.*

The Story of Mr. Camp: From Bedside to Administrator's Office

Ruth Purtilo, Ph.D.

This is the way the world ends, not with a bang but a whimper . . .
—T. S. Eliot

THIS is an account of my involvement as an ethics consultant
with a patient whose story goes on and on. Usually, an ethics
consultant sees the end of a consultation. Occasionally, however,
there is no discrete ending. This is not a neat case: the patient was
difficult to work with; no one could engage him in reasonable discussion; the treatment staff continued to be conflicted about what to do. I
was unsure of my own role, and I do not know what eventually happened to the patient. Still, this is a case I want to describe.

Act I

Scene: The Surgery Department

The story of Mr. Camp begins on a crisp October day . . .

Ruth Purtilo is Henry Knox Sherrill Professor of Medical Ethics and Ethicist-in-Residence at Massachusetts General Hospital, Boston.

Mr. Camp was a sixty-eight-year-old man who lived alone in a blue-collar area of the city. He was admitted to the surgical unit of Middletown Community Hospital after falling from a footstool in his apartment. He was apparently trying to reach a can of peas on the top shelf of his kitchen cupboard when his footstool broke, throwing him to the floor. The noise alerted Mrs. James, a neighbor, who called the police after she had knocked on his door and received no response. The police broke down the door and found Mr. Camp unconscious on the kitchen floor. He regained consciousness on the way to the emergency room.

An x ray determined that he had sustained a longitudinal double fracture of his left femur, the large weight-bearing bone in his leg. It also revealed a hip joint severely damaged by arthritis. The surgeon decided that a hip replacement was not indicated. Mr. Camp was taken to the operating room for reduction of his fractured femur.

Prior to surgery, Mr. Camp seemed confused about what had happened to him but otherwise appeared oriented. No one doubted his competence to give consent for the surgery. The social worker contacted Mrs. James, who had called the police. She said that Mr. Camp had lived alone in his apartment for approximately twenty years. He was reclusive and had become increasingly withdrawn and belligerent after his brother had died six years earlier. She knew of no other relatives and said she was actually quite afraid of Mr. Camp because sometimes he would pace the corridors of the apartment building, stopping in front of the doors of other apartments but never knocking on the door or trying to turn the knob. He went out for groceries and beer often. He shouted profanity in his apartment, presumably to himself; she believed he did not have a telephone. The local neighborhood grocer and tavern owner said they knew almost nothing about his private life in spite of the fact that they saw him in the shops almost every day. The grocer told the social worker that he thought Mr. Camp was a "mean old bastard."

Following surgery, Mr. Camp seemed more confused than before. Several times he told nurses that he didn't know why he was in prison and thought he should have an opportunity to see his lawyer. A CT scan was performed to rule out brain damage resulting from the fall. All reports were negative. He received daily physical therapy treatments and made very good progress with a walker. He talked daily about getting home.

At the end of three weeks the surgical resident raised the question in a team meeting of whether Mr. Camp was ready for discharge from the hospital. The physical therapist and the chief resident (the physician in whose care Mr. Camp had been since surgery) believed that he was physically able to return home but would not be able to remember to keep the weight off his leg and would almost certainly reinjure it. They thought he needed nursing home placement as a temporary safety measure. Others disagreed, thinking he could do well at home with a visiting nurse. The judgment that it was better to send him to a nursing home prevailed at that meeting. The social worker agreed to talk with him about the staff's concern about his safety.

When Mr. Camp heard the gist of the social worker's discussion, he swore loudly and said he would "walk out if they tried to send me to a nursing home." Further attempts to raise the subject with him were to no avail. Later that day, in physical therapy, he purposely put weight on his healing leg and said, "See! I'm ready!" When the therapist pled with him not to do that, he defiantly stood on the leg again. The decision was made to try to keep him in the hospital for a while to instruct him further about the danger of reinjuring his leg.

On a Wednesday an ethics consultation was requested. It took place during the Friday morning regularly scheduled team meeting, one week after the possibility of discharging Mr. Camp had first been raised. Prior to the team meeting I spoke with him. He thought I was his sister and said that it was a shame he had to go through so much to get me to come visit him. When I tried to explain that I was a member of the hospital staff, he began to swear under his breath. I believe he knew he had made a mistake, that I was not his sister. He turned his back to me and would not talk.

Was an ethics consult appropriate at this juncture? I believe so. The resident who requested the consult said he didn't know if the problem was "exactly an ethical problem," but "each of us is using ethical reasons to support our points of view." When asked for an example, he replied, "Well, the ones who think he can go home are talking about his right to independence, and the ones who want him to go to a nursing home are talking about their duties and responsibilities." He added, "We usually work pretty well together, but once in a while things heat up. We seem to be at an impasse on this one, and the thermometer is rising."

At the meeting I outlined four areas that are useful to examine in complex ethical problems:

1. The clinical efficacy or futility of any proposed interventions.
2. The patient's (and/or family's) preferences.

3. The patient's quality of life at present and probable quality of life as a result of the proposed interventions.

4. The proper role of cost considerations, laws, and existing policies in the current situation.[1]

The team members quickly identified the areas they believed were the sources of their ethical problem: (1) disagreement about the clinical efficacy of the proposed treatment (sending Mr. Camp to a nursing home temporarily) and (2) disagreement about his competence to express his preference. All agreed that he was extremely upset at the thought of going to a nursing home. I told them about my conversation with him, and the social worker agreed to investigate the possibility that he might have a sister somewhere.

The Ethical Conflict

I asked the group to identify which professional duties and responsibilities should guide their decision making in this case. They agreed that their primary duty was to do what was best for the patient clinically, to try to prevent harm to him. In addition, several staff members, those who thought he was not mentally competent to be sent home alone, emphasized that he needed to be protected from himself. If he went home, he would probably reinjure his femur and might well be worse off than before. On the one hand, they wanted to honor his preference to be at home; at the same time, they were worried that to do so might lead to harm. The patient's right to autonomy was a concern for them.

This ethical impasse was caused by a conflict of principles. The health professionals knew that to engage in one course of action, consistent with their duty of beneficence and nonmaleficence, might prevent them from honoring his autonomy. The two principles led in divergent directions. To choose one might compromise the other. At this level of deliberation, the staff was experiencing an ethical dilemma:

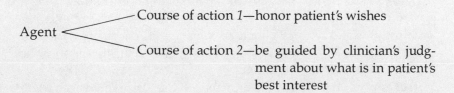

Agent
— Course of action 1—honor patient's wishes
— Course of action 2—be guided by clinician's judgment about what is in patient's best interest

They were attempting to reduce the dilemma by persuading Mr. Camp that entering a nursing home was in fact best for him.

Reasoning about the Conflict

In the second step of the consultation we addressed approaches to weighing these ethical principles. Should autonomy govern? Now the discussion focused on a difference of opinion about Mr. Camp's competence. This was a sensitive point, a topic around which accusations began to mount. It turned out that no one liked Mr. Camp very much. The staff saw him as a cantankerous old man, belligerent at times and altogether unpleasant. Some thought his periods of "confusion" were deliberate manipulations; others believed he was sometimes confused (though always distasteful). The chief resident, himself under a lot of strain from the overloaded service, had said to one of the nurses who wanted to send Mr. Camp home that the nurses were always willing to get rid of the patients they did not like and "fight like hell" to keep pleasant patients in-house. The nurse, of course, told this to her colleagues, and the battle lines were drawn. The chief resident apologized at the meeting, saying he hadn't meant exactly what he'd said, but it was time the nurses took his opinions seriously. He said they acted as if they knew better than he about the patient's mental status. The physical therapist said that although he agreed with most of the chief resident's judgment calls, he had to disagree with that statement about the nurses. Mr. Camp seemed to slink into the shadows as the dynamics of the team came center stage for fifteen minutes. I realized that no rational discussion would ensue about ethical principles until we could solve the problem of the patient's mental status. When I said this, the chief resident agreed and suggested having the consulting psychiatrist see Mr. Camp. Since Mr. Camp's insurance would allow him to stay a few more days, they and he could profit from more attention to the plans for his discharge.

Reassurance

The third step was to reassure the staff that as far as I could tell each person was trying to do what was best for Mr. Camp, though further attempts to help him return home were in order. I encouraged them to use what they had learned in this meeting in their further work. The chief resident said he would request a psychiatric consult. The social worker, nurses, and physical therapists said that they would each try to watch more closely for signs of his ability to function alone at home and would continue to search for alternatives that would allow him to be cared for at home. All seemed relieved that his stated preference to go home was not going to be dismissed lightly. I offered to return for the next team meeting if they thought it would be beneficial. They said it probably wouldn't be necessary. I left the consultation with the feeling that a better course of action (in this case constraint while gathering more relevant information before discharging Mr. Camp) would be forthcoming.

Act II

Scene: The Surgery Department Continued

I almost always follow up on an ethics consultation, so I called the chief resident three days later. He said that a psychiatric consult was conducted the day after the team meeting. The psychiatrist found Mr. Camp "agitated and only questionably competent," with cognitive symptoms suggestive of early Alzheimer's disease. He also recommended that Mr. Camp's medications be assessed closely to minimize any side effects that might be decreasing his orientation or increasing his agitation. He believed that Mr. Camp could have "lost ground" during the stress of his injury and hospital stay. Meanwhile the staff had concluded that Mr. Camp was a "sundowner," a term applied to people who become less oriented as the day goes on.

The staff, the resident added, seemed to be coming to more agreement about sending Mr. Camp to a nursing home temporarily with the goal of returning him home when the injuries were healed. I asked what Mr. Camp thought about this course of action. The resident replied, "Well, we haven't told him outright, but we're preparing him in that direction and are confident he is feeling much more favorably about going to the nursing home. We plan to discharge him next week if we can find a place. I plan to talk with him myself this evening and expect everything to go smoothly. By the way, we haven't found that sister. Thanks for your continuing concern in this issue and for your help." On some occasions I follow up with a visit to the patient, too. When I suggested this to the resident, he replied that it might not be appreciated by Mr. Camp. I agreed and let it go at that.

Intermission

I forgot about Mr. Camp. It is not the first time I have taken the gratitude of the team as an adequate sign that an ethics consultation helped to solve a problem. It's not the first time and probably won't be the last that my assessment was wrong.

Act III

Scene: The Administration Office

On December 23, almost two months after the original consultation, I was called by a hospital administrator to ask if I would attend a meeting in his office regarding an institutional problem of a patient who had "wreaked havoc" in the hospital. He had not talked with the health professionals yet and wanted to check with me first about my availability. When I asked what my role would be in such a discussion, the administrator responded he would like me to be an objective observer and participant because everyone else present had been so close to the situation that he feared the patient in question might have become the victim rather than the beneficiary of our services. As he described the problem, I realized that the patient must be Mr. Camp. The administrator confirmed that it was and was surprised to learn that I had been involved in Mr. Camp's case before. (I do not write in the patient's medical record, so word about my consultation is dependent on having the ethics consultation reported by the physician or other health professionals who call me.) I told the administrator that the first round of consultation had involved some team problems that might better have been handled by a person formally skilled in group dynamics. I questioned whether the present meeting required an ethicist's presence or was more strictly an administrative matter. He said he wasn't sure but would like my attendance if possible.

When I entered the conference room, I greeted the eight team members I had met with in October. Also present was the hospital administrator who had called the meeting, the psychiatrist, a second social worker, the director of nursing, the head of security, the director of the patient's representatives service, the hospital's chief legal counsel, and the quality assurance committee chairman. Everyone in this large group looked "in extremis" on this day before Christmas Eve.

In a nutshell, from what I could gather, the following had taken place: The evening after my follow-up call, the chief resident decided to take Mr. Camp's "favorite" nurse and a social worker in to talk with Mr. Camp. As the resident began to broach the subject of nursing home placement, Mr. Camp swore at them and turned his back. None of the three could induce him to talk though each tried to reassure him that their goal was to return him to his home as soon as possible.

That same night, about ten o'clock, Mr. Camp tried to climb over the bed rail, which had been raised for the night. He probably would have succeeded in doing so if a nurse had not come by at that very instant. She called to him to get back into bed and started toward him. He swore that he was being held against his will and threw a water glass at her, narrowly missing her forehead. She called for help. It took two nurses and an orderly to push the now screaming and writhing Mr. Camp back into bed from his tenuous position straddling the rail. His shouting continued for about an hour in spite of attempts by several nurses and the resident on call to calm him. He was given a tranquilizer and tied down to the bed. Eventually, he fell into a fitful sleep.

Apparently things went downhill from there. The next day a nurse was helping him to the bathroom with his walker. Suddenly he swirled around and threw the walker at her. She was thrown off balance, let go of him momentarily, and he fell. He fractured his left hip. She was not injured but was very shaken and asked not to be assigned to treat him again. She offered to resign but was encouraged to take a few days off, was offered counseling, and the next week returned to work. Mr. Camp, now confined to bed because of his hip injury, became increasingly difficult to handle. In the next three weeks, he often tried to strike nurses and three times was successful. He threw a bed pan filled with urine and feces at a nurse's aide. He bellowed almost continuously. He threw food at everyone. He was tranquilized often and often put into restraints. Requests were made by the surgical service to transfer him to the psychiatric unit, but the hospital does not have psychiatric beds for long-term patients. The psychiatrist was sympathetic with both the hospital's and the patient's dilemma. He judged that Mr. Camp's mental status had deteriorated considerably and believed he should be placed in an institution for the chronically mentally ill, where he could be followed over a period of time to better evaluate his mental status. Nonetheless, many of his caregivers continued to believe that he was "more mean or frustrated than sick" because he had moments and even hours at a time of great lucidity. Two social workers worked diligently to find placement for him in either a nursing home or an institution for the chronically mentally ill. Because of his now bedridden status, questionable Alzheimer's disease, and violent outbursts, no nursing home would accept him; because of his diagnosis he did not qualify for placement in state-owned institutions for the mentally ill. He did not have enough insurance to qualify for a private mental institution.

In short, by December 23 everyone who had contact with him despaired for, despised, or feared Mr. Camp. In spite of this, almost every health professional was still trying to provide him with good care. Some nurses refused to enter his room, but on every shift some were willing to provide him with the care he needed. The nursing department administration was sympathetic and tried to accommodate as well as possible to this difficult situation for the staff.

When Mr. Camp's wrists showed signs of beginning skin breakdown—he never seemed to stop struggling against his restraints—the restraints were removed permanently and the security guard was called whenever a nurse or other health professional had to enter the room. At first the security staff complied willingly, but after two weeks they became weary of being on call. On several occasions they took so long to come that a nurse would enter the room with just another nurse or staff member. It was on one such occasion, after Mr. Camp had been calling for help for five minutes, that the head nurse had gone in with only another nurse. Mr. Camp grabbed the head nurse and placed a stranglehold on her, trying to choke her. She broke away, gasping. She called her supervisor, then her husband, then the patient representative. She was crying. Her husband called the hospital lawyer and threatened to sue the hospital. That was December 21.

At the December 23 meeting, everyone looked tired. I thought about how much attention the care of one patient can require from a well-trained and well-meaning staff in a well-organized and well-administered institution. The issues, as laid out by the administrator, were these: A patient with violent, combative behavior has been in the hospital for nearly three months. He has almost no money left, no relatives, and apparently no place to go where the staff believes he will be well cared for and safe. He does not need an acute-care hospital bed. He is costing the hospital approximately $520 a day, none of which the hospital can ever hope to recover. He must be extremely miserable. From the staff's point of view he is a dreaded, even hateful, patient.[2] The lines of support within each hospital administrative unit have been working well: nursing administration has ensured that Mr. Camp's nursing care continues while supporting individual nurses' legitimate fears and hesitation; the surgical department administration has tried rotating the residents to provide relief to the beleaguered chief resident and to give Mr. Camp the benefit of new residents who have built up less resistance to having to face him; the psychiatric service has provided whatever treatment they can to Mr. Camp and has offered support to the team to deal with their stresses; security services have only reluctantly refused to provide ongoing protection for health professionals having to go into the room, stating that "unfortunately we are not a twenty-four-a-day police protection service." Individual employees have felt loyal to the hospital and appreciated the administrative support. For example, the nurse who had been placed in a stranglehold was trying to prevent her husband from pursuing a lawsuit because she believed her loyalty to her job might appear to be less than what she actually feels. Other nurses who had submitted incident reports following Mr. Camp's assaults on them played down the seriousness of the assaults when called by the quality assurance committee. The chief resident stops by to see Mr. Camp even though he no longer is officially responsible for his care.

It was the hospital's legal counsel who initially called the hospital administrator. Only by working backward, touching base with two clinical departments (surgery and psychiatry), nursing, physical therapy, occupational therapy, social work, and, finally, security, did one person, the hospital administrator, eventually reconstruct the full extent and duration of the problem.

What is the role of an ethics consultant in this type of institutional quandary? It is rare, I believe, for an ethics consultant to be asked to help with a system-wide "fire out of control." Nonetheless, I believe that the three R's for an ethics consultation (which I have outlined elsewhere[3]) apply: To *recognize* the principles inherent in a problem, to *reason* about and weigh these principles, and to *reassure* the participants that key ethics issues have been considered thoroughly. The ethics consultant also is a resource for further deliberation, as this case shows.

Because Mr. Camp's care involved many units of the hospital, *institutional* values and principles needed to be taken into account. Two values guiding institutions are justice and efficiency.[4] Each individual in the institution should be able to anticipate equitable treatment, and the institution should run smoothly so that its varied functions can be as fully realized as possible.

"Each individual" in this situation includes each patient, each health professional, and all others. Each employee deserves consideration. The institution has a moral responsibility to provide protection for each employee when harm related to the job is present.

I called attention to the magnitude of the ethical problem. The goals of supporting Mr. Camp's good (optimum patient care), the health professionals' good (job satisfaction and protection from physical harm), and the institution's good (efficiency, satisfied employees, good public relations, high-quality patient care) could not all be met in this case. Mr. Camp could be given adequate care, and health professionals could be protected only at the great *in*efficiency of keeping Mr. Camp in an expensive hospital bed, spending inordinate administrative time to protect and rotate staff, providing security, and holding extensive meetings about how to proceed.

Which principles and values should govern in this complex situation, and why? Everyone, including the administrator, would acknowledge that the primary function of a hospital is to provide optimum patient care. But to safely provide Mr. Camp with optimum care was simply too costly in terms of staff hours, staff suffering, and consumption of institutional resources. The present situation could not continue.

Everyone agreed that Mr. Camp would be better off in a long-term care facility other than the hospital. I asked if Mr. Camp had expressed any more wishes to go home. Apparently, he no longer talked about going home, but his apartment was still being held for him, thanks to Mrs. James and the social worker who had worked out a plan for keeping the apartment. The staff very much wanted him to have a placement that would at least move him in the direction of being home, if that would ever be possible. Finally, the psychiatrist offered to make a call to collect on an old favor that was owed her by the staff in a highly respected community mental health agency for both the acute and chronically mentally ill. A weekly visit by a physical therapist to the agency could be arranged. The psychiatrist was confident she could talk the agency's administrator into admitting him. Everyone agreed that she should try, though we knew this "spot welding" approach to the issue would not help to resolve a similar problem if it arose again.

I reassured the staff. I believed we had chosen an ethically justified course of action. The administrator thanked me for my input and said how grateful he was I had come.

But I left this meeting feeling let down. I was not certain that Mr. Camp's care was going to be better. At the same time, I did not know what else could possibly be done. I sympathized with the nurses and others who were struggling to find a solution. It seemed as if we all were having to settle for the lesser of the evils. We had discussed how we could prevent this kind of long and difficult situation from repeating itself. Toward this end we agreed to let each other know when problems seemed to be getting out of hand, especially if they began to involve more than one department and the usual lines of reporting and support were not working. Since I am involved in many different units of the hospital, it was agreed that I could be a key person to notify. I could then identify the nature of a burgeoning problem and talk with the administration. Enthusiastically I agreed. Later I worried about whether I was the appropriate person to be assuming that type of reporting relationship to the administration. What about patient confidentiality? What about the trust relationship I had built up with the lay staff in the hospital—would they become more hesitant to utilize my services?

On January 7, Mr. Camp was transferred to the institution for the mentally ill. Everyone breathed a sigh of relief. Mr. Camp did not resist at all. In fact, he seemed relieved.

Act IV

Scene: Medical Department and Home

On February 11 I met the social worker in the corridor. She said, "Mr. Camp is back." I asked why. She said he had had an acute psychiatric episode the past weekend. The administrator at the private facility put Mr. Camp in an ambulance and returned him to us. He was admitted to our acute-care psychiatric unit and three days later was transferred to a medical floor. The social worker said she thought he would be sent home fairly soon. No nursing home was interested in taking him. His femur was healed to the point where he could put weight on it. His hip fracture was healed. That day I went to see Mr. Camp. I just wanted to have some contact with him again. He was sleeping. He looked very small in the hospital bed. I left.

The next day the social worker called me to say that they were having a discharge planning meeting and they'd like me to attend. "You and I are the two people who have had the most opportunity to know this man's long history," she said. Again, I agreed to attend. None of the people who had been present at the last meeting about Mr. Camp were present except the social worker and me. The social worker had been trying diligently to return Mr. Camp to his apartment: Mrs. James said she had worked out a plan for her neighbors to help her keep an eye on him; a home health aide would visit daily at first; Meals-on-Wheels would assure a meal; a visiting nurse could be made available once a week for four weeks. Everyone was worried about whether he'd be able to function at home.

Four days later, February 16, Mr. Camp arrived at his apartment. The social worker went along, and Mrs. James was present. The apartment was dirty, probably just as he had left it the day he reached for the can of peas, but Mrs. James had put fresh sheets on the bed. When the social worker asked Mr. Camp if he was glad to be home, he said, "No."

Some months later I again met her in the corridor of the hospital. "Mr. Camp?" I asked. "I don't know," she replied, shrugging her shoulders. "You know, once people leave here it is difficult to keep track of what happens to them. What are you ethicists doing about the Mr. Camps? I tell you, I get discouraged trying to find places for people like him to go. Some days I feel like I just can't continue putting people in places where I am not sure they will be OK."

An older woman, shabbily dressed, brightened up when she saw the social worker and called to her by name. The old woman said, "I was looking for you! I was wondering if you could . . ." I moved on down the corridor.

Notes

1. This is the organizing framework for analysis of ethical problems in A. Jonsen, M. Siegler, and W. Winslade, *Clinical Ethics* (New York: Macmillan, 1982).

2. Several articles have appeared in recent years addressing the problems of "hateful" patients. One treatment of the subject is Raymond Lande's 1989 article, "The Dangerous Patient," *Journal of Family Practice* 20(1):74–78.

3. R. Purtilo, "Ethics Consultations in the Hospital," *New England Journal of Medicine* 311(1984):983–6.

4. Rawls argues for the primacy of justice while conceding the persistence of efficiency as a value of institutions. See John Rawls, *A Theory of Justice* (Boston: Harvard University Press, 1961).

This is a short essay, but there is much
to contemplate within it about the role of the
ethics consultant and about human nature. It is a gem.

The Power of Denial

John D. Golenski, S.J.

THE power of denial has always astonished me. Over the years of consulting with physicians and hospital ethics committees, I have never encountered a case where denial about the patient's condition or prognosis and, to some extent, about the feelings thus generated was not present. It becomes the stuff of ethics consultation when the primary participants' degrees of denial vary and interfere with clear, value-directed decisions. Some years ago, an unusual pediatric case illustrated the power of this mechanism of defense.

A little girl was born to a working-class family in the Midwest eight years ago. Her parents, David and Pat Andrews, decided to name her Vivian in honor of her maternal grandmother, Mrs. Berger. Little Vivian was their third child, following a boy, Denis, seven, and a girl, Diane, four. Four months after birth, while Pat was out shopping for groceries with her other children, grandmother Vivian was baby-sitting her namesake. Mrs. Berger had put the baby down for a nap and had herself fallen asleep in a living room chair with the newspaper on her lap. It was a hot summer day.

Pat returned with groceries and kids, gently woke her mother, and then went into the baby's room. She found Vivian cold and still. She attempted CPR but only knew the adult technique from seeing it on

John Golenski is a member of the Bioethics Consultation Group in Berkeley, California.

television. Mrs. Berger had the presence of mind to dial 911, and the paramedics arrived quickly and carried out a full resuscitation.

Dave arrived at the hospital, having been called at his construction job. Baby Vivian was now connected to a breathing machine (ventilator), still alive but not showing any signs of higher central nervous system function. The chief of service of the pediatric intensive care unit (PICU) had assumed direction of her care and had directed various affiliated professionals to work with the family. Unfortunately, the family lived in a town where the local sheriff's department was untrained in and unsophisticated about sudden infant death syndrome. Hence, grandmother and parents were grilled about possible physical abuse. Some of the relatives, over the days of initial hospitalization, also implied that responsibility for Vivian's condition rested with Pat or Mrs. Berger. Denis and Diane also displayed predictable signs of a stress reaction.

Throughout Vivian's hospitalization, Dave and Pat were absolutely consistent in refusing even to consider discontinuing ventilatory support, though Vivian showed no signs of improved neurological function. On a few occasions, when Vivian's Aunt Meg openly questioned the rightness of prolonging the child in this state, the parents, especially Pat, angrily accused her of not loving Vivian enough or not trusting in God enough.

The PICU staff were concerned that the family was not coming to terms with the baby's condition. They employed every strategy they knew that might break the family's denial. The physicians, nurses, respiratory therapists, and social worker were united in their belief that Baby Vivian should be removed from artificial respiration and allowed to die.

As the weeks wore on, the family resisted all efforts to work with them except when the staff relayed clinical information about Vivian's condition. A major battle ensued when the PICU medical director informed them that Vivian was no longer an appropriate admission in the PICU, that she must be placed in a long-term-care facility and that her medical care consequently would not be as intensive. Dave was especially angry when told that Vivian was not ever expected to improve.

As frequently happens in tertiary-care units, the staff's concern and sense of urgency about a decision for Vivian waned considerably when finally she was transferred to a skilled nursing facility (SNF). Before transfer, Vivian received a tracheostomy, a surgically created opening in the front of her neck, connected via tubing to her ventilator. Her pediatrician worked out a long-term treatment plan in consultation with the PICU medical director and the SNF's medical director.

The nursing staff of the SNF became particularly committed to Baby Vivian. They usually provided care to elderly patients, and the presence of a baby generated an unusual intensity of concern and involvement. For the first six months, Dave and Pat visited often, occasionally bringing in their other children. Mrs. Berger, at least by report of the social worker assigned to the case, never recovered from the loss. She found it difficult to visit, and when she did, she would hover over the crib weeping and murmuring to the baby.

Since the SNF was not accustomed to infant patients, the medical director tried to keep the family pediatrician involved in the case. Not too long after Vivian's admission, the family dismissed their pediatrician because of his repeated requests to review the decision to continue ventilatory support. They subsequently found another doctor who was willing to assume responsibility for Vivian's case.

The SNF's record showed that over the seven years of the baby's stay, her parents' visits became less and less frequent until the routine was literally a yearly visit by Dave alone. The record also showed a change of pediatrician every two years or so, with increasing expressions of frustration over the family's intransigence in the pediatrician's progress notes. It became a sad joke among the SNF staff that Vivian was their baby. They seemed to be the only consistent persons in Vivian's life. Her grandmother, Mrs. Berger, died a few years after Vivian's admission, and Dave and Pat did not allow Vivian's siblings to visit.

Why such long-term cases result in a request for an ethics consultation at some point is often unclear. In the case of Baby Vivian, it is probable that her appearance became increasingly unacceptable to the staff. The staff and the pediatrician became quite impatient with the case at about the same time. Somehow Dr. Sanderson, the pediatrician, had managed to remain involved for a little over two years. When she began attending Vivian, she made clear to Dave that she expected some decisions would need to be made in the next few months. Months had grown into years, and Dr. Sanderson's patience was wearing thin. Staff distaste was turning into anger, especially since a number of very sick but conscious patients had recently been refused admission to the SNF because beds were unavailable. Vivian's body had grown into a grotesque, contorted shape. She showed no signs at all of higher mental function, lacking even responsive eye movement. Whenever she was taken off the ventilator, she was entirely unable to breathe on her own.

Although the staff's negative feelings were running high, Vivian had never, in her years of care, had one bed sore. Her physical care was exemplary.

Dr. Sanderson had requested a family conference one month before her call to me. Dave had come alone to her office and, as always in the past, categorically refused any consideration of discontinuing his daughter's ventilatory support. Dave said he believed that every doctor's attempt to remove Vivian from the ventilator had been the result of pressure exerted by the insurance company. He insisted that with proper medical care Vivian would eventually improve and wake up. He often described miracle stories of people waking from coma after years. Dr. Sanderson maintained her composure in the face of his angry threats to sue her or bring criminal charges against her if she reduced the level of any of Vivian's care. She informed Dave that he would have a very difficult time finding yet another pediatrician if he dismissed her from Vivian's case and that she was committed to caring for the child even though she did not believe that Vivian would ever recover. She assured him that she would never discontinue or significantly alter the level of Vivian's care without his and Pat's consent. Dr. Sanderson was convinced that she could work with Dave if she could maintain his trust.

Dr. Sanderson and I had met at a recent medical conference sponsored by the local hospital where she admits her acute-care patients. My colleagues and I provide ongoing consultation to the Institutional Ethics Committee of the hospital, and she had heard some of her pediatrician friends describe the ethics case rounds that we regularly hold in the intensive care nursery. She told Dave about me and about the ethics committee and asked if he would agree to an informal review of Vivian's situation. He was willing at least to continue to discuss Vivian's case with Dr. Sanderson but refused to participate in an ethics rounds.

In response to Dr. Sanderson's request, I suggested that we hold special ethics rounds in the SNF with a few members of the nearby hospital's ethics committee. The hospital and the SNF had a close working relationship, and most internists in the community admitted patients to both. Dr. Sanderson and the SNF director of nursing, May Shields, were happy to hold the rounds there. In fact, Ms. Shields asked if some of her nurses could attend.

At noon on Wednesday of the following week, Dr. Sanderson convened the first ethics rounds to consider the case of Vivian Andrews. The consulting neurologist for the hospital was present, as well as May

Shields; Betty Manstein, Vivian's social worker; Amelia Troy, her primary care nurse; and several other nurses. Dr. Gary Torrens and Margaret Saunders, R.N., co-chairs of the hospital ethics committee also participated. The case review followed the usual format for such consultations with a careful recounting or the relevant information about Vivian's case. As I anticipated, the early discussion was a venting of the caregivers' feelings of frustration, anger, and guilt. After reviewing Vivian's history and confirming that the neurologist's diagnosis was still of a child in a persistent vegetative state, I allowed discussion to range far and wide. I suggested that Dr. Sanderson speak with Dave and try to persuade Pat and the family to come in for a conference soon. After informing the family that the team was reviewing Vivian's case at ethics rounds, Dr. Sanderson was advised to invite the parents again to attend follow-up rounds, scheduled for two weeks later.

I learned from May Shields that a great deal of discussion had occurred among the nurses during the intervening two weeks. Vivian had become almost an institutional mascot, with everyone presuming she had always been there and *would* always be there, silent and unaware. Having the rounds shook loose the perceived ordinariness of her presence. The initial discussion again focused caregivers' attention on the extraordinary reality of a child whose body grew over seven years with no coincident mental development. Vivian was a physical presence with no discernible inner life but with great importance in the lives of the staff. In a real sense, the staff began the process of accepting the eventual death of Vivian, and various signs of initial grief began to appear. By the time of the second rounds, the nursing staff had at least incorporated the notion that Vivian might not remain in the unit indefinitely and that she would die sometime in the near future.

Dave and Pat were skeptical of the process of the rounds but agreed to visit Dr. Sanderson in her office to hear about the results of the deliberation. They continued to refuse to participate in the rounds. Dr. Sanderson believed they were intimidated by the thought of having to state their position to a group of strangers. At the second rounds, the process of considering what was best for Vivian was dramatically clearer and less erratic than during the first rounds. Curiously, there was as much emotion, but the expression of feeling was more directed, focusing on the anticipated loss from Vivian's departure from the SNF and on her eventual death.

It was decided that the family would be asked if they would meet with Dr. Sanderson in Vivian's room rather than in the pediatrician's office and that they would be informed that Vivian was not an appropriate patient for the SNF. Dr. Sanderson and Ms. Manstein would prepare a discharge plan for Vivian's care at home. The family would need to go to the SNF frequently for a few weeks to learn how to care for Vivian, especially how to manage her tracheostomy.

The family reluctantly agreed to meet with Dr. Sanderson in Vivian's room, though they did not understand why they had to go to the SNF to assist in plans for her continued care. Dr. Sanderson had told Dave only that Vivian needed some changes in her care routine and that she thought it would be a good occasion to apprise them of Vivian's status and relate the results of the ethics rounds to them together. The family was predictably stunned by the notion of providing Vivian's care at home. Dave protested that she needed the protection of the nurses' expertise and vigilance, as well as the ready availability of medical care. Dr. Sanderson had consulted with the family's insurer, and she was able to insist that the SNF beds were appropriate for individuals needing more continuous nursing assistance. She added that the insurance company believed there was no longer a good reason for Vivian to be receiving round-the-clock skilled nursing care.

I had suggested to Dr. Sanderson that in conferring with the family this time she should not even broach the question of stopping therapy. Though everyone who participated in ethics rounds agreed that termination of ventilatory support was the best course of action to follow with Vivian, it would not help to provoke an adversarial relationship with the family by initially insisting on this position.

Although we anticipated that Vivian's family would eventually see the reality of her condition after she had returned home, no one expected the brief period of training in the SNF to affect them as much as it did. Our goal in asking their cooperation with the ventilator training was simply to ensure that Vivian could indeed be cared for safely at home. Everyone was surprised when Vivian's father asked Dr. Sanderson for a meeting after he and Pat had attended just one session of training.

Dr. Sanderson agreed to meet with Vivian's parents in her office the next afternoon. Dave told her that he and Pat had discussed Vivian's situation and had decided that it was cruel to prolong her life. He acknowledged that it had been impossible for either of them to accept that she would never wake up again and to deal with their own sense of responsibility for her condition. Somehow, they said, spending time with her at this point brought them face to face with their daughter as she was now.

Dave and Pat spent some time with Dr. Sanderson discussing what would be best for them, their other children, and the staff in discontinuing Vivian's ventilatory care. They chose not to be present when Dr. Sanderson actually removed the ventilator but requested time to bring their other children to the SNF to say good-bye. They also understood that the nurses who had, in a real sense, adopted Vivian would need their own time for farewells.

When Dr. Sanderson gathered the staff to apprise them of Vivian's status, they were at first astonished by the rapidity of the family's decision, and then they were shocked to realize that Vivian actually would die very soon. It seemed advisable at that point to shift the focus of this third meeting from the actual decision and the family's involvement or lack of involvement to an airing of the staff's feelings, especially their surprise and grief. We moved to a general discussion of individual staff members' feelings for Vivian and about her. There were tears, periods of silence, and contradictory comments about the parents' irresponsibility in prolonging her dying and for discontinuing care so abruptly.

A time and day were set by Dr. Sanderson a few days hence in order to give the family a chance to visit. By the next day, when Dave and Pat brought the children in, the staff were supportive and helpful, allowing the parents as much time as they needed. Pat and Dave had invited their minister to help them with a service, and this seemed to make the transition clear and definitive.

After the family's departure, the staff gathered in Vivian's room. So much had been said before that words were scarce. It seemed appropriate to be together with Vivian in silence. Eventually, one of the nurses, hearing her name called over the PA system, moved toward the door. As she passed the bed, she touched Vivian's forehead. This gesture seemed to invite others to touch Vivian before leaving. One by one, the staff—nurses, respiratory therapists, the dietitian, the social worker, and Dr. Sanderson—moved to the bed and made physical contact with Vivian's body. Some touched her hand; one kissed her forehead; most touched her head.

Finally, I was left in the room with Dr. Sanderson and the nurse on Vivian's shift. While the nurse gently held Vivian's head, Dr. Sanderson removed the ventilator tube connected to Vivian's tracheostomy. After several shallow gasps, Vivian was still. After a moment, both Dr. Sanderson and the nurse were quite businesslike in removing all of the other tubes and devices from Vivian's body. For the first time in more than six years, Vivian was separated from technology, machines, and fluids. She had not been separated from human caring.

After Dr. Sanderson left, returning to her duties and responsibilities to other patients and to the solitude of her own conscience, I remained in Vivian's room with her nurse, Joan Casperino. Joan washed Vivian's body and began the process of wrapping her in preparation for an autopsy, which is required by law. Pat and Dave had left a fur-covered Paddington bear with Vivian, and Joan included the stuffed animal in the body bag. Before she entirely closed the container, she tucked in at Vivian's breast a large, bright day lily, which she took from an arrangement that had been sent to another patient. As I was about to leave, Joan asked me for a hug. It seemed a gentle irony that this woman whose work for months had afforded the semblance of physical comfort to a child who could not experience or understand it asked so little comfort for herself.

Dr. Sanderson phoned some days later to talk over what had occurred, what she had done, and what she had heard from the family. She had attended a public funeral, as had some of the nursing staff. Pat and Dave had again expressed their thanks for her help and their sorrow that Vivian's dying had been so long. With time and the inevitable changes in staff, the image of Vivian will fade until there will be only an institutional memory of that child who was here so long and whose parents were unable to accept the inevitable.

Certainly, the ethical questions in Vivian's case were not unusual. Many patients in SNF's across the country are hovering in a twilight state just short of death, their lives prolonged on machines with indiscernible benefit to them, because of family, physician, and staff denial. At the same time, each such "case" is the unrepeatable stuff of a human life, not reducible simply to cognitive function or potential for cure. Vivian Andrews was a human body with very few human functions remaining, but nonetheless, with the complex net of relationships focused on her, a human being. Her functional demise had, of course, occurred when she was four months old. However, her death—an event mediated by the perceptions, choices, and actions of others—took place seven years later.

Howard Brody's is a complex case, intelligently
and satisfyingly written. It is a fine exegesis of
how two ethics consultations, many weeks apart, did
and did not affect the progression of a difficult case.

Did It Make Any Difference?
Ethics Consultation in a
Community Hospital

Howard Brody, M.D., Ph.D.

POLITICS and communication difficulties are hardly absent in university hospitals, but they may manifest themselves in somewhat
different fashion in a community setting. This alters, to some
extent, the factors that an ethics consultant must attend to in a community hospital. The following case may illustrate some of these issues,
even though the lessons yielded may easily be applied to university
hospitals as well. I will first relate the story of the patient's illness during
the course of hospitalization, then add the story of the two ethics consultations that occurred during that course, and finally offer some critical
reflections on the consultation process when looked at retrospectively in
relationship to both the case and the setting. It will soon be clear that this
is not offered as any sort of success story; the case has been chosen
deliberately to illustrate problem areas and missed opportunities.

The Case of Mr. Samuel Stevens

Our community has four hospitals, all of which have some medical
school affiliation and serve as sites for training residents and medical

Howard Brody is Associate Professor of Family Practice and of Philosophy at
Michigan State University in East Lansing, Michigan.

students. The hospital on whose ethics committee I serve is located in the poorer section of town, and many black and Hispanic families prefer it. When Mr. Samuel Stevens, a sixty-eight-year-old black retired custodian, showed up in the emergency room of one of the other hospitals on January 31, complaining of increasing shortness of breath and ankle swelling for the past day, an ECG monitor showed an abnormal rhythm (bigeminy) and a blood test indicated a toxic level of his digitalis medication. Clearly, he needed to be admitted, and he and his family wanted him to be hospitalized in their neighborhood, resulting in a cross-town transfer and admission to the combined intensive care and coronary care unit.

Mr. Stevens had been in ill health for some years. A little more than a year previously he had suffered a heart attack. He also had high blood pressure and had been treated for tuberculosis many years ago. In the past he had been both a heavy smoker and, for a shorter time, a heavy drinker, but he had quit these habits in the past several years.

The patient was admitted under Dr. Wang, an internist who was on call for admissions that evening but who had not had prior contact with the patient or his family. Dr. Wang did the bulk of his work in two other hospitals (including the one at whose emergency room Mr. Stevens first entered the system). It was his routine to make rounds very early at this hospital so that he could get on to see the majority of his patients at the other two sites.

Mr. Stevens was initially managed for digitalis toxicity and congestive heart failure, and the possibility that he had had another heart attack was investigated; but nevertheless he worsened. He developed shallower respiration, decreasing consciousness, and slurred speech; all of these seemed to point to a stroke or some other neurological insult in addition to his heart problems and some degree of kidney failure. By February 2 he was unable to breathe on his own and had to be placed on a mechanical ventilator. At this point Mr. Stevens clearly needed closer attention than Dr. Wang could provide, given his busy practice elsewhere, so Dr. Wang consulted Dr. Farrah, who was a specialist in pulmonary medicine and who managed a teaching service with residents assigned to it. This meant that a physician would be on call twenty-four hours a day to respond to any additional crises. Although many practitioners would simply have turned the case over to Dr. Farrah's service at this point, possibly looking in once a day to justify continuing to collect a daily fee, Dr. Wang did not do that. He continued to make rounds early each morning and continued to interest himself in the patient's plan of care.

With a lung specialist now on the case, a good deal of the management was directed at the breathing problem, although a CT scan of the head was done and seemed to indicate an area representing a possible new stroke, thus explaining the loss of consciousness. But interest turned to the possibility of a lung tumor or some other underlying lung problem. The x rays appeared suspicious for some sort of mass near the windpipe; two bronchoscopies (looking into the lungs with a lighted flexible tube through the windpipe) were done and also were thought to be suspicious, but no firm diagnosis was made. A surgeon was consulted about the possibility of a direct surgical approach to look into the mediastinum, the area around the windpipe. Also, after two weeks or so with a flexible tube in his throat attached to the ventilator, the patient would need a tracheostomy instead, to assure that the ventilator would continue to work appropriately. By mid-February the patient had shown no ability to breathe when not attached to the ventilator, but he had shown a very slight improvement in mental function; occasionally, he was able to look at people and to follow simple commands. Unfortunately, he also was quite agitated and tried regularly to pull at the tube in his throat. A strong sedative was required to prevent his doing damage to the life-support equipment, and accordingly it was hard to assess his true level of consciousness.

Mr. Stevens had a wife and three daughters, who visited regularly but had had little contact with the physicians and no say in the treatment decisions. Dr. Farrah decided to call a family conference on February 13; together with his resident, Dr. Strong, he met with the family and a nurse in the ICU. (Dr. Wang, who had made his early morning rounds as usual, was not there.) The purpose of this meeting was to tell the family about the poor progress to date, to warn them of the likelihood that Mr. Stevens would not do well, and to emphasize the need (as perceived by the pulmonary team) to make a firm diagnosis of the underlying lung problem. The family accepted this information passively; they offered no particular responses, and apparently nothing by way of response was requested or encouraged.

On February 16, Dr. Wang came late in the day, when things looked rather worse; Mr. Stevens's blood pressure had dropped precipitously, and he required a special drug intravenously to restore it to satisfactory levels. Dr. Wang now held his own meeting with the wife and two of the daughters. He also indicated his pessimism about recovery, and he asked for and received a specific response from the family: they agreed to a do-not-resuscitate (DNR) order for Mr. Stevens. (This was their response to the bleak prognosis presented by Dr. Wang; there was no evidence that Mr. Stevens himself had ever expressed any wishes on the matter prior to hospitalization.) This meeting was apparently quite a stressful one for the family; Mrs. Stevens, who also had high blood pressure, was found to be quite hypertensive afterward and had to be taken to the emergency room for observation. Mrs. Stevens later admitted to a social worker that she had some guilt feelings about the hospitalization, wishing she could have prevailed on her husband to seek care earlier. She had also asked one of the elders in their church to visit him.

These two family conferences showed some lack of concordance between the two principal physicians. Dr. Wang, the official attending, was becoming quite pessimistic about Mr. Steven's chances, but he also was unwilling to consider removing the respirator; he felt that this would probably be illegal. A DNR order seemed to him to be a proper recognition of the bleak prognosis and moreover, one that he knew to be well within the bounds of legal practice. Dr. Farrah was better informed about withdrawing mechanical ventilation and knew that there was no legal barrier; he also shared Dr. Wang's view of the poor prognosis. From Dr. Farrah's viewpoint, the time for decision on continued respiration was rapidly approaching. It seemed to make little sense to go ahead with the surgical intervention (tracheostomy and mediastinoscopy) if the respirator might be removed soon afterward anyway. There seemed to be two logical courses of action: decide that the prognosis was poor in any case and consider withdrawing the respirator, or go all-out to establish a firm tissue diagnosis and then decide on treatment based on that diagnosis. The lack of response to treatment, the patient's long smoking history, and the suspicious x rays all combined to make Dr. Farrah and his residents consider the possibility of lung cancer. If the family initially resisted the suggestion to turn off the respirator, the clear knowledge that Mr. Stevens had cancer might be enough to help them to see the futility of further treatment.

This divergence of views soon became academic, however, because an unexpected development occurred: Mr. Stevens became somewhat more alert and was better able to respond to the presence of visitors and to follow commands, though he continued to be unable to communicate any sort of complex thought. In this circumstance, none of the physicians could generate much enthusiasm for discontinuing the ventilator, even though the DNR order was continued in force. In case calorie deprivation might be a factor in the poor breathing response, Mr. Stevens was begun on full intravenous nutrition. Finally, on February 26, the situation was stable enough to allow the surgeon to do the tracheostomy and mediastinoscopy, but no tissue diagnosis of cancer or any other specific condition resulted.

By March 1, Dr. Farrah had become more pessimistic about the value of continued respiratory support for Mr. Stevens and asked for another family meeting. (A new resident, Dr. Berliner, was now on the case, as the residents rotated every four weeks.) The family was now more forceful in requesting continued active treatment; they were impressed with the fact that there had been some improvement in consciousness and no longer shared the physicians' assumption of an inevitably fatal outcome. Dr. Farrah suggested that they schedule a weekly family–physician conference during his usual time for morning rounds. A further outgrowth of this session was that two of the daughters were found to be having difficulty coping with recent events, and the liaison psychiatry team in the hospital was consulted and asked to provide additional family mental heath support.

The month of March was occupied mostly with continued efforts to improve nutrition and to see whether Mr. Stevens could be weaned from the ventilator. Weekly family conferences were held. Since the weaning process went poorly at first, and the family continued to insist on ventilator support, the discussion was now expanded to include eventual nursing home placement, as indefinite hospitalization would not be feasible. No local nursing home was equipped to handle a ventilator patient, and the only available facility seemed to be a home located in a city sixty miles away. However, Mr. Stevens's insurance and Medicare status was such that the nursing home would not accept him until all of his present hospital coverage was exhausted—in effect, he would have to be hospitalized for 105 days before a new insurance benefit would become applicable and make him eligible for the nursing home! By contrast, if he could somehow be weaned from the ventilator, local nursing homes would then be feasible.

These family conferences also helped to clarify the family's attitudes and concerns. Outwardly, all discussion dealt with future planning for continued life support and nursing home care. But some other issues were occasionally revealed, often to the nurses or the social worker. Mrs. Stevens and one daughter noted that they "still believed in miracles." Also, Mrs. Stevens had expressed concern that her husband had moved away from the church in recent years, whereas she had remained very devout. Her view was that it would be a bad thing for her husband to die now because he had not yet had a chance to "get right with God." If he became more alert and came back into the fold of the church, his death subsequently would be something that she could accept much better.

On March 30, the patient was less responsive mentally, but there were some indications that the nutritional program was paying off. It might finally be possible to disconnect the ventilator and allow Mr. Stevens to breathe on his own with an oxygen tube attached to his tracheostomy site. Intensive discussions were held that day between the family and Dr. Weichsel, the third in the series of residents to work with Dr. Farrah on the case. Perhaps for the first time, the decision regarding the ventilator was put in concrete terms of Mr. Stevens's level of function, instead of whether or not a "miracle" was likely. Presented with the prognosis that Mr. Stevens would never be mentally more alert than he was now, respirator or no respirator, the family finally came to an agreement that he would probably not wish to be kept alive in that state indefinitely. (Of course, this state did not allow him to "get right with God" in any meaningful way as his wife had wished.) They agreed to a trial off the respirator to see if he would breathe on his own. If he did, local nursing home placement would be sought; if he deteriorated again, they accepted the implications of the DNR order, that he would not again be reconnected to the ventilator. Dr. Wang was again not present, but he added a progress note to the chart—his first to address explicitly the overall management plan, as opposed to the day-to-day treatment issues—agreeing that the patient should be weaned from the respirator and then "we can exercise our DNR . . . we can let nature take its course." On the other hand, if the patient did well off the ventilator, he hoped there might still be some gradual neurological improvement. He still harbored doubts about the legality of this course and indicated a desire to consult with the hospital attorney on the matter.

On April 4, both Dr. Weichsel and Dr. Wang reaffirmed the family's acceptance of the weaning/DNR plan; by now Dr. Wang appeared to be convinced that he was in no legal jeopardy. On April 5, the weaning from the ventilator was carried out successfully. As this measure eliminated the need for continued intensive care, Mr. Stevens was transferred to a regular hospital room on April 7, having spent sixty-six days in the ICU to this point.

At 1 A.M. on April 8, a nurse found Mr. Stevens without respiration or pulse. According to the DNR order, no resuscitative efforts were made. Dr. Wang was called, and he asked that the resident on call for Dr. Farrah's service be requested to examine the patient and pronounce him dead. Two of the daughters, contacted by the nurses, came in to view the body and then went to tell their mother. Later that morning the nurses spoke with Mrs. Stevens on the phone. She appeared collected and accepting of the event; she did not wish to come to the hospital.

Two Medical Ethics Consultations

As a family physician and teacher of medical ethics at a medical school that is affiliated with many community hospitals, I am asked approximately a dozen times a year to consult formally on an "ethics case." One feature of these consultation requests is highly predictable: they will arrive in my office either when I am out of town or when I am just about to go out of town. Mr. Stevens's case was no exception. I was out of town on February 12, when a nurse called from the ICU to report that Dr. Wang had written an order on the chart to request an "ethics consult." The secretary who answered the phone was new and simply put the message in my mail slot, not realizing that this was a matter of some urgency. (Our hospital has a general policy that consultants, to maintain staff privileges, must respond to a request within 24 hours.) Accordingly it was not until February 16 that I first saw Mr. Stevens.

Our program in medical ethics has provided consultation service for approximately nine years, since well before the formation of hospital ethics committees in our community. When this hospital began its committee three years ago, it took a while to get the group "up to speed" in terms of basic knowledge and protocol. By the time Mr. Stevens had been admitted, however, it was decided that the committee ought to become more active in case consultations, at least on an on-the-job-training basis. I negotiated for the opportunity to continue to involve the staff of the university in these consultations as well, for our own internal training needs. Therefore, when I came back to town and tardily discovered the phone message, the first order of business seemed to be to assemble the appropriate consultation team. The group that was pulled together included, besides me, a physician and a nurse from the hospital ethics committee and a visiting professor in our medical ethics program.

We planned to meet in the ICU, review the chart, see the patient briefly (having been forewarned that he was unable to communicate), and then discuss the case with any available nurses and residents. We arrived in the late morning, after Dr. Wang had made his early rounds and about the time that Dr. Farrah's team often came by. Knowing how Dr. Farrah's team often became the "dumping ground" for ventilator-dependent patients initially admitted by attendings who did not have their own resident coverage, I assumed that Dr. Farrah was actually managing the case and that Dr. Wang had signed the order as a formality.

We also encountered a fairly common problem in requests like this. The request for consultation referred vaguely to "decisions around life-sustaining treatment." It was not at all clear exactly what questions we were being asked to address. We plunged ahead into the chart, however, in the hopes that later discussions with nurses and residents, and perhaps with Dr. Farrah, would clarify the matter for us.

The chart was again fairly typical for this setting. The physicians' progress notes dealt almost entirely with day-to-day concrete management issues. There was little mention of long-range plans or for the rationale behind treatment. Neither was there any mention of family wishes or reactions in the physicians' notes. Usually nurses' and social workers' notes are more informative on these matters; but as of February 16, even these sources were fairly uninstructive. The family's usual daily visit, as it happened, generally occurred in the afternoon, and so no family members were present to interview directly.

My usual plan of facing cases like this one is first to review all of the available data, including both medical information and preferences of the patient or family, relevant to the decision. Next, possible treatment or management options are listed. Finally, the options are weighed according to some stated ethical values or principles. If one and only one decision seems to be defensible, that course is recommended and a rationale given. (The old saws "An ethics consultation should analyze the issues but never give answers" and "There are always two sides to an ethical question" seem to me to be usually incorrect. Consultants are frequently brought into a case because there are important practical issues to resolve. The case itself, not some prior dogma, should determine whether specific advice or a particular recommendation is appropriate.) If the case seems to be a "toss-up," alternative rationale for different courses of action are provided, and the responsible parties are advised to choose among them. Finally, I convey these findings or recommendations to the physicians by some combination of face-to-face discussion, brief summaries written directly into the progress notes, and a fully detailed typed summary usually running three to four pages (which cannot be transcribed and placed in the chart until at least 24 hours after the consultation). Especially when residents or students are involved, I try to mention some journal articles or other key references.

Looking only at the available data, we immediately discovered two significant gaps. We saw no mention of a full neurological assessment in which any physician's view of the long-term prognosis for recovery of consciousness or mental function was recorded. And we saw no mention of the family's wishes or desires or of whether they had been asked what the patient's desires or wishes were if he had ever expressed any.

We next tried to list and assess the medical options. (As three of the members of the consultation team were physicians with experience in such cases, it was easy to assume this role and also to risk offering advice or criticism that was not properly within the scope of "ethics.") We saw three major options: (1) to make a decision now that ventilator support was not in the patient's interest and recommend its cessation, (2) to await the definitive tissue diagnosis on cancer and then make a decision about appropriate level of treatment, or (3) to continue respirator support under the assumption that if the prognosis is really as bad as it appeared, other organ systems would eventually fail, in effect taking the decision out of the physicians' hands.

All of these options presented difficulties. Option 1 ran into the gaps in the data base noted previously. Option 2 made the assumption that, first, a definite diagnosis would be made and, second, that that would somehow change the sort of management that seemed appropriate; but both of these assumptions were questionable. We thought there was a good chance that mediastinoscopy would fail to yield a tissue diagnosis, as bronchoscopy had already done. Moreover, cancer in the mediastinum is almost impossible to treat successfully with either surgery or radiation, and all lung cancers respond very poorly to chemotherapy; so knowing whether or not the patient had cancer seemed unlikely to change anything substantial in the management plan. (We assumed that whether the patient or his family would favor life prolongation probably had more to do with the long-term *neurological* outlook—whether he could think and communicate, breathe on his own, or resume activity—whereas the dominant physicians seemed to be more prone to look for a diagnosis relevant to his long-term *pulmonary* outlook, which seemed unlikely to reverse his ventilator dependence in any substantial way.) Option 3 led to the problem that the time it might take for other organ system dysfunction to supervene, or for the prognosis to become clear by default, might be unacceptably long. It is of some minor interest to note that these *medical* judgments about the case, made on February 16, seem in retrospect to have been quite accurate.

When the time came for conclusions or recommendations, we found ourselves unable to apply ethical values or principles, for the simple reason that the data base was inadequate. Accordingly, all of our recommendations were for further data gathering and recording in the chart. Here we added our suspicion that fragmented communication between the attending physician and the pulmonary consultant might have contributed to the perceived difficulty of the case; and we suggested that before sitting down with the family and laying out options for their consideration, it would be wise to make sure that the medical team agreed among themselves on prognosis and treatment choices. We offered our later services if assistance was needed with the family conference but left it to the medical team to sort out their own communications for themselves.

Before we left the ICU we were able to speak briefly with Drs. Farrah and Berliner as they came by on rounds, and they basically confirmed the impressions we had gleaned from the chart. I then wrote a brief summary progress note and excused the other members of the consultation team while I sat at the dictaphone and dictated the full consult. I added a promise that we would look in on an ongoing basis to see if further help was needed.

It was only as I was leaving the ICU after completing this dictation that Dr. Berliner made a chance remark that answered our first question—why we were consulted originally. He observed that Dr. Farrah was quite willing to consider turning off the respirator if matters did not improve soon, but he was frustrated because Dr. Wang thought that this would be illegal. Apparently, Dr. Wang had ordered the consultation by way of confirming his own impression. I hurriedly returned to the dictaphone and added a note to the written consultation to clarify our view that no ethical or legal barriers stood in the way of discontinuing a respirator, so long as either the patient or the family requested this and the medical team felt that continued support was no longer offering the patient any benefit. (It is my habit not to offer legal advice but instead to summarize the prevailing views from the literature in medical ethics, which, of course, includes legal opinion.) Only at this late stage of the consultation process did I discover belatedly exactly what question the consultation request had been intended to answer.

When our group visiting the ICU the next day and the day after, we found out that several changes had occurred. First, Dr. Wang had written the DNR order, and, second, Mr. Stevens was becoming a bit more alert. We did not find that either of the pieces of missing data (neurological prognosis or family's wishes) had been addressed in the chart. We did, however, receive the impression from the nurses and from Dr. Berliner that as long as there was a DNR order and Mr. Stevens seemed to be making some neurological improvement, things were going along in a satisfactory manner, and additional advice or input from us was unnecessary. We accordingly ceased to follow the case for a time.

Our next contact with this case occurred many weeks later, on March 29, when Dr. Weichsel phoned me to ask for a repeat consultation. Somewhat surprised to learn that this patient was still in the hospital and that no definitive decisions had yet been made, I asked whether it would suffice to arrange for a consultation the next morning. Dr. Weichsel agreed and noted that, to his mind, the problem now was that all of the physicians were agreed on the patient's poor prognosis, yet the family was resisting the need to confront this fact and was totally fixated on placement in a skilled nursing home.

I then turned to the task of assembling our team for the consultation the next morning; the group that eventually came together included a nurse from the hospital ethics committee, a philosopher from our academic program, and another visiting professor. In focusing on the arrangements for this meeting, I failed to clarify some important issues with Dr. Weichsel. I assumed that, as this was a reconsultation on the same patient, Dr. Wang, who had initiated the consult request the first time, had also agreed to this second consultation. I also assumed that our mission was to review the chart, update ourselves on the patient's medical condition, and update our list of options and recommendations accordingly. Both of these assumptions turned out to be erroneous.

On the morning of March 30 we met in the ICU and reviewed the chart since February 16. We noted that the neurological improvement had plateaued for the past two weeks, with Mr. Stevens occasionally making eye contact and occasionally squeezing a hand when asked to do so but showing no signs of any increased level of function. We also noted that other medical problems had surfaced, especially infection and anemia. The chart now better documented the concerns of the family and tended to validate Dr. Weichsel's statement that they were concerned only with nursing home placement and were not responding to efforts to get them to confront the seriousness of the prognosis.

We concluded at this point that little had really changed since we made our suggestions on February 16. Neither the DNR order nor the decision to continue treatment as long as the patient was improving neurologically had really solved anything, and the search for the diagnosis of any underlying lung lesion had not paid off as hoped. Although there was more in the chart about the family's wishes and views, there was still nothing like a comprehensive statement of the long-term neurological prognosis. And we found on inquiry that the lack of agreement between Drs. Wang and Farrah continued; indeed, it now was discovered that Dr. Farrah's team had asked for the present consultation in large part out of frustration because Dr. Wang was not (in their minds) dealing adequately with the patient's poor prognosis. Dr. Wang had not approved our return to the case. We were thus being maneuvered into a position to be used to oppose the wishes of the attending physician.

Once again, Drs. Farrah and Weichsel were on their usual daily rounds, and Dr. Wang was not available. After discussing the situation with the nurses and physicians, we decided simply to restate some of our earlier suggestions in a second note. To us, the ethical question was whether the family, acting as the appropriate surrogate decision maker for Mr. Stevens and having been adequately informed about the prognosis, believed that continued ventilator support counted as a net benefit for Mr. Stevens. But before we could raise this question to the family in a meaningful way, it was essential that Drs. Wang and Farrah reach an agreement on the likely prognosis and the available options for care at various levels. We therefore suggested that improvements of communication on the medical side be the first order of business, followed by frank discussions with the family. We reasserted our view that there was no ethical or legal barrier to discontinuing the ventilator if the view of the family was that it offered no benefit to the patient— that is, that life prolongation itself, in the absence of any functional improvement, would not be construed as a benefit.

As I had done before, I went to dictate the formal consultation note. Since listening to somebody talk into a dictaphone for ten minutes is a fairly unilluminating activity, I suggested that the other members of the ethics team might leave. It was only after I had completed the dictation that the social worker, who had arrived toward the end our discussion, mentioned that the Stevens family had been waiting in the ICU lounge for forty-five minutes to speak to us, at Dr. Weichsel's request. Dumbfounded and rather irritated by this news, I asked Dr. Weichsel if he had wanted us, as part of our consultation process, to interview the family, and if so why he had not made this clear over the phone. He replied that he had not actually expected us to do this but had assumed that we might want to talk to them and thought it safest to be sure they were on hand. He had told them that some "ethics people from the university" were coming by to "see what sorts of decisions might be made" about Mr. Stevens.

I now had to decide what to do about this. On the one hand, I wished not to have an interview with the family by myself, without the input of the rest of the ethics consultation team, as this would seem to defeat the whole purpose of the team process. On the other hand, I felt that it would be highly impolite to ignore the family after they had been waiting patiently and also highly disrespectful and counterproductive if the impression were somehow given that decisions were being made without their input. I decided that respect for the family would have to win out over ideal process and went to talk with them.

I was introduced by the social worker to the wife and three daughters. I briefly explained how our group viewed the consultation process and reminded them that the attending physicians were still the medical decision makers and would necessarily have to have input into any major decision about Mr. Stevens's care. I then went on to explore their understanding of his prognosis and of the options available for them to consider. All of them voiced an understanding that his failure to improve was not encouraging and that even with continued respirator support there was a high likelihood of further medical complications. They seemed to understand that it was quite unlikely that he would recover any more function than he now displayed. They informed me further that he had never personally expressed any wishes about the desirable level of care in such circumstances, but they had doubts about whether he would want to be maintained in this level of relative incapacity. At this point it appeared that progress was being made in the direction that Drs. Farrah and Weischsel seemed to be hoping for.

But then one of the daughters made a forceful statement in favor of continued aggressive treatment, alluding to the need for faith and "hoping for a miracle" which had been noted previously by the social worker. It was striking that the other family members had been subdued in expressing their views, whereas this daughter was quite dynamic and almost cheerful. In short, she carried the day; no one seemed to wish to oppose openly what she had said, even though they had just a few minutes earlier been saying things that directly contradicted this outlook.

I made some tame comments that Drs. Wang and Farrah would probably be meeting to be sure they had looked at all realistic options and would then be back in touch with the family, and I made my departure. I felt on the one hand, that I had successfully defused any possible misunderstanding about what the ethics squad might be doing to their loved one behind closed doors. On the other hand, I had uncovered further evidence of a split in opinion within the family, which could be as hard to resolve as the apparent split within the medical team. I left quite pessimistic about reaching any sort of resolution in this setting, and my pessimism was reflected in the final line of the consultation, offering reassessment at a later date if asked but not offering to follow along on a daily basis as we had before.

There were no further requests for input from anyone involved. I learned a couple of weeks later that the patient had died. It was not until doing a detailed chart review at a later date that I found out all of the details of Mr. Stevens's last days between March 30 and April 8.

Critical Discussion

Mr. Stevens's travails in the hospital lend themselves to critical analysis in some depth. I will first look at how the medical team managed the case and then turn back to how the ethics consultation process was conducted.

Simplifying matters for a moment and assuming that Drs. Wang and Farrah fundamentally agreed on the goals of therapy, I would characterize the medical management of Mr. Stevens's case as falling into three phases. The first, lasting from admission on January 31 until about February 28, consisted largely of a search for underlying diagnoses. During this phase, it seemed to be agreed that it was highly unlikely that Mr. Stevens would live long or would recover any significant degree of function; but it also seemed that this information by itself, in the absence of a firm diagnostic label, was insufficient to yield acceptable conclusions about the appropriate level of care. (For example, the extended and ultimately vain search for a pulmonary diagnosis could be viewed as seeking evidence for a malignant process within the chest—not because that could be treated but simply because knowing that Mr. Stevens had cancer would make the eventual withdrawal of the respirator more palatable both to Dr. Farrah's team and to Mr. Stevens's family.)

The second phase, lasting from about February 28 to March 30, was predicated on two facts: (1) a firm diagnosis of serious underlying disease could not be obtained; and (2) neurologically, Mr. Stevens had improved to some slight degree. In this setting, withdrawal of life support, beyond the DNR order that had already been entered, was not seen as acceptable (especially given the family's wishes). Instead, the practical aim of therapy was to improve the patient's pulmonary status to the point where he could be weaned from the ventilator. (The stepped-up nutrition program was the clearest part of that effort.) The backup goal, should the primary goal prove impossible, was to gain admission to a skilled nursing facility where Mr. Stevens could be cared for while on the ventilator. Both the primary and the backup goal required careful medical manipulation; for example, no nursing home would accept Mr. Stevens in transfer if he had any active infection, so sources of sepsis had to be rigorously identified and proper antibiotic therapy administered.

The last phase, during the first week of April, consisted of what I have elsewhere called (without any intent to be disparaging) a "managed death."[1] It was based in turn on some new facts: (1) Mr. Stevens had indeed improved to the point where weaning was possible for the short term, although later deterioration was highly probable; (2) he had ceased to improve in any other functional or mental capacity; and (3) the family was finally becoming more resigned to his poor prognosis and that he might not leave the hospital. Dr. Wang, in his statement of the therapeutic plan on March 30, made it reasonably clear what was intended, using only thinly veiled terms such as "exercising our DNR" and "letting nature take its course." Mr. Stevens would be weaned from the respirator, and all of the medical team realized that this weaning would probably be only transient and that his underlying condition would make it impossible for him to breathe for long on his own. But by the combined fact that he was DNR status and that he no longer needed the respirator, a twelve- to twenty-four-hour stable period would be sufficient to justify transferring him out of the ICU. Once on the regular ward, he might die suddenly, unobserved; or if he was observed to be getting worse, the team could justify refusing to reconnect the ventilator as contrary to the intent of the DNR order. But it was essential to the medical team's and the family's comfort with this course of action that it not be *called* "managed death" or anything of the sort. Officially, the patient had improved and no longer needed ICU care; this was simply a trial to see "whether he could make it on his own." (Of course, the chance that he *could* make it on his own was not zero; and if this happened, the medical team could claim that this was their goal all along—though it is doubtful that they would have been truly happy about it.)

Similarly, removing the respirator (in the full foreknowledge that it would not be reconnected) was not *called* "discontinuance of life-prolonging therapy" or anything of the sort; it was "weaning." Basically, the medical team and the family made a decision on March 30 to limit the level of life-sustaining treatment that Mr. Stevens would receive, but they maintained the comforting fiction that no decision had really been made—the DNR order had been on the chart since February 16, and the weaning was a natural outcome of recent improvements in the patient's own ventilatory capacity.

From the viewpoint of the ethics consultation team, there were many features of the medical management of the case that were suboptimal. Almost throughout Mr. Stevens's long hospital course (Dr. Wang's note of March 30 being a major exception) the physicians concerned themselves solely with the day-to-day management issues and never addressed the long-term prognosis or plan. As part of this limited vision, they expended much time and effort in the search for a pulmonary tissue diagnosis without asking whether this information would really have any bearing one way or the other on the patient's treatment. Faced with the need to make some sort of ethical choice, they secured a DNR order and then acted as if that single order answered all of the other ethical questions. At least on Dr. Wang's side, unrealistic fears of legal impropriety seemed to cloud all discussions of ethical choices. Finally, communication overall was poor. Drs. Wang and Farrah seldom communicated directly, and most communications with the family were aimed at giving them desired information, rather than learning from them their own thoughts and wishes. (Although I have introduced this case as typifying in many ways the problems of ethics consultation in community hospitals, I would nevertheless suggest that each of these deficiencies could equally well have been encountered in a university hospital setting.)

What the ethics consultant would have wanted, ideally, was a medical team that was unfettered by unrealistic legal fears and had optimal communication both internally and with the family. As soon as the basic features of the case were known (such as the stroke and the cardiac condition), the team would have evolved a comprehensive management plan, including both treatment modalities and further diagnostic maneuvers that would substantially alter treatment. The patient's prognosis, both for survival and for return of function, would have been accurately predicted; if this were impossible, the management plan would have specified the length of treatment necessary before the prognostic information would reveal itself. After treatment had proceeded for that length of time and the prognosis still remained poor, the team would then, in collaboration with the family, look at options for limiting or ceasing life-prolonging treatment. In sum, there would be more rational planning at each stage of the process, and the need for decisions, as well as the basis for the decisions, would be openly communicated.

My point here is simply that whenever a consultant is called into a medical case, the consultant's first reaction is to state, "Here's how I would manage this case if it were up to me"; and indeed, this information is often precisely what the consultant is being asked to provide. But the consultant is *not* the physician managing the case. In the final analysis, the most successful consultant is one who knows not only his or her own preferred logic but also the "logic" of how the case is unfolding in the hands of those who are responsible. If the proper ethical information or advice can be framed within that latter "logic," all is well. If the case management logic is too flawed to admit sound ethical input (as often happens when communication is poor and prognostication issues have been avoided), then the disparities must be squarely faced in a manner helpful to the attending physician and the house staff. Just saying, "I would have done this differently" is rarely helpful.

I have looked at what might have been wrong (or right) with the management of the case, but what about the ethics consultation? In retrospect that process seems to have been afflicted with some major flaws. Given that poor communication was one of the difficulties identified at both consultation sessions, could not our team have done a better job of facilitating that communication? My failure to speak directly with Dr. Wang on either occasion and my inability on both occasions to get clear on exactly what I was being asked to do before I arrived for the consultation indicate the extent to which I exacerbated rather than helped to resolve that communication problem. It seems, with benefit of hindsight, that I was more engrossed in the unfamiliar task of covening the consultation team according to our new protocol than I was with what was needed for the best resolution of the case at hand. Moreover, I fell prey to the fact that I personally knew Dr. Farrah and his residents fairly well and did not know Dr. Wang at all; under those circumstances it was easy to treat him as a peripheral character when he should have been the central focus.

Given the facts that the medical team was proceeding according to their own logic, which the ethics consultations did not directly address, and that the ethics consultation process itself was less than ideal, can we reconstruct the impact, if any, that the consultations had on the outcome of the case? As already noted, the chart gives virtually no evidence that any of the recommendations were followed or even acknowledged; indeed, no mention at all of the first consultation appeared in the physicians' subsequent progress notes. It might appear at first glance that the consultations did nothing to aid in the care of the patient.

My reading is that more was accomplished. The first consultation occurred just before the DNR order was written. Although the DNR order by itself does not constitute a plan of care, it does signal that the issue of prognosis was being addressed and that communication with the family about possible future scenarios was occurring at least at some level. The second consultation immediately preceded the approach that I have called "managed death" and may have helped the medical team to realize that continued life-prolonging therapy was not the only defensible option. Moreover, the family interview that occurred as part of the second consultation appeared at the time only to cement the internal disagreements, but in retrospect it may have helped the process of confronting some family members with the bad news because they agreed soon afterward to the plan not to reconnect the ventilator.

I cannot attribute these developments solely to the ethics consultations themselves because the readiness to request a consultation suggests that the medical team is open to a rethinking of its actions. In this regard, requesting ethics consultation may be something like seeing a psychiatrist: admitting that one has a mental problem and that one needs outside help may ultimately be more therapeutic than any specific thing that the psychiatrist says or does once therapy begins.

Whereas the ideal logic of the case, seen from my standpoint, might have called for earlier and crisper decision making, the logic as seen by the medical team may have better reflected the actual tempo of Mr. Stevens's case as it unfolded. There was enough prognostic uncertainty—the unlooked-for improvement in neurological function in mid-February and the eventual ability to come off the ventilator—and enough uncertainty within the family to derail any attempt at an earlier decision. True, with better two-way family communication, the issues of special concern to them might have been identified and worked through earlier, and the family might have ended up less optimistic about the skilled-nursing-placement option, which occupied much of their attention through March. But it is also possible that the slowness of reaching the final decision, and the ambiguity that surrounded that decision, simply reflected what the parties most directly involved were prepared to face at any given time.

In the end, Mr. Stevens's case was managed jointly by Dr. Wang, Dr. Farrah, and the house staff. Dr. Farrah was the more reluctant partner, and he might have wished for an earlier limitation of treatment; but Dr. Wang's pace of decision making may have better reflected the needs of the family (ironically, because Dr. Farrah's team was in more regular communication with the family than was Dr. Wang). The medical team requested two ethics consultations and very selectively took from those consultations the bits of information or counsel that happened to fit the logic and the pace of the case as it was unfolding in their hands. And of course, that is precisely how the responsible physician ought to approach consultation advice, whether from a cardiologist, pulmonologist, or ethicist. The inability of the consultant to force advice on the attending physician (particularly in a community hospital setting) is very clear in this case, and in the final analysis it seems the soundest base on which to build the consultation process.

Finally, there were gaps in communication, and the ethics consultation was objectively correct in pointing them out. But the process itself could have been better used to plug some of the very gaps it complained of. Maybe that is not ethics in any strict sense, but it is helpful. And striving to be helpful is not an inconsiderable aim for the process of ethics consultation.

Note

1. H. Brody, *Stories of Sickness* (New Haven, Conn.: Yale University Press, 1987) 161–70.

This last essay is the most personal in the book. Ron Cranford writes about his involvement with the medical care of his dying mother-in-law, Betty. Cranford was not a formal consultant to Betty's physician, but he assertively brought to bear the knowledge and case management skills of an ethics consultant. This is an appropriate final essay in a book intended to reveal the personal as well as the conceptual aspects of being an ethics consultant.

The Role of the Ethics Consultant in Personal Ethical Dilemmas

Ronald E. Cranford, M.D.

ALMOST all ethics consultants will be involved at some time with ethical dilemmas involving their family, their friends, or themselves. In fact, given the pace of advancing medical technology and the dramatic increase in ethical problems created by this technology, most consultants may be confronted by multiple ethical dilemmas involving their own lives.

Ethical dilemmas requiring the assistance of an ethics consultant or an ethics committee vary significantly in their complexity and manner of resolution. Some—for example, when the ethics consultant has been faced with the same problem many times before—are easy to resolve. The consultant, drawing on his or her experience, can often be of considerable value to the health care professional who may be facing the dilemma for the first time. For example, a competent patient with end-stage chronic obstructive lung disease is now completely ven-

Ronald Cranford is Associate Physician in Neurology at Hennepin County Medical Center, Minneapolis, Minnesota.

tilator-dependent. Numerous attempts to wean him from the ventilator have failed. Knowing that stopping the ventilator will result in his death, the patient nonetheless says that he wants to die and asks only to be kept comfortable during the dying process. An attending physician who has never faced this dilemma before may be filled with anxiety and doubt and may have many questions about the medical and moral legitimacy of following the patient's directions. When should withdrawal be carried out? Should the patient be given medication for suffering (e.g., air hunger, a distressing symptom in which a patient gasps continuously for air and feels as if he is suffocating) when and if it occurs? When is giving a large dose of morphine to alleviate suffering equivalent to killing the patient (a form of active euthanasia)? How does one draw the line between giving doses of medication adequate for relieving suffering and doses that may be lethal?

At my institution, an acute-care hospital, it is not uncommon for competent patients to request withdrawal of ventilator assistance, which will almost certainly lead to their death. This has been one of the more frequent types of ethical dilemmas brought to the attention of our ethics committee. Over the last seventeen years of our committee's existence, we have handled at least fifteen such cases. We have never gone to court and have almost always satisfactorily resolved these dilemmas by using decision-making mechanisms within the institution.

Other dilemmas are more difficult to resolve. A family may be deeply divided about the appropriate treatment for their loved one. For example, a son who has been out of contact with the patient and family for years may differ with his siblings about stopping treatment. He may say, "The rest of you can do what you want, but I'll never kill my mom." Disagreements within the family can be the result of long-standing intrafamilial disputes of twenty or thirty years duration. They can be exceedingly difficult, if not impossible, to resolve in a short time at the bedside of a dying patient.

Some consultations are not only intellectually difficult; they are emotionally taxing as well. The balance between maintaining professional demeanor and expressing personal feelings is sometimes precarious. There are those who say that ethics consultants should never show emotion and should always remain detached. I don't believe that, and I don't think most experienced ethics consultants do either. One of the most highly charged situations, at least in my experience, is the unexpected and tragic death of a child. Working with parents who are about to lose a child, and thinking of how we would feel if this were happening to us, can leave ethics consultants totally drained emotionally and physically.

Or: dealing with the parents of a previously healthy child who has accidentally aspirated a hot dog into the trachea only a few hours before is an experience that no one will ever get used to. To look the parents in the eyes and tell them that their child's brain is totally destroyed when the child looks perfectly "normal" (although appearing asleep and on artificial life-support systems) is something that a health care professional can never forget no matter how many times he or she does it. A neurologist-ethicist like me is often called in on these cases, not only to determine that brain death has occurred but also to talk with the parents.

Thus, when an ethics consultant is presented with an ethical dilemma involving his or her own family or friends, some questions inevitably arise. Will my emotions cloud my professional judgment and wisdom? Will it be harder or easier for me to do what is appropriate when it involves my loved ones? Some would argue that physicians or ethics consultants should never be asked, "What would you do if you were in my situation?" or "How would you treat your loved one in a situation like this?" Others, including me, would argue that these may be legitimate questions in some situations. Would you, as a health care professional and ethics consultant or member of an ethics committee, treat your loved ones differently from the way this patient is currently being treated?

In May 1987, my wife's sixty-four-year-old mother, Betty, developed generalized weakness while at her home in Winter Park, Florida. A chest x ray revealed a large mass in the lung; a biopsy showed cancer. Betty's face was swollen because the tumor was pressing on the main vein draining blood from the face (superior vena caval syndrome). The long-range prognosis for this type of tumor is extremely poor. Many patients die within three to six months, even with surgery, radiation, and chemotherapy.

Bud, my wife's father, died of lung cancer in 1981, also at the age of sixty-four, nine months after the initial diagnosis. As the disease ravaged Bud's body, he experienced the typical symptoms of terminal cancer: fatigue, weight loss, nausea, anorexia, and air hunger.

In 1981, the doctor in Florida caring for Bud had assured him and the family that, when the end was near, Bud would not suffer needlessly. But when Bud was imminently dying, this physician (like so many other physicians) was reluctant to give his patient adequate pain medication to relieve his suffering from air hunger. Bud experienced a substantial amount of needless suffering in his dying hours.

It was never clear why this physician allowed Bud to suffer in this way. There are so many *bad* reasons why doctors don't adequately treat pain and suffering in the dying patient that it is sometimes hard to select the one that seems uppermost in a physician's mind: fear of killing the patient with too much medication; concern about legal liability, which often clouds all sense of compassion and common sense; simply not taking enough time to know the patient's needs; fear that the physician's decision-making autonomy may be eroded by allowing individual patients to decide how much medication they need; or fear of causing addiction in a terminally ill patient who will be dead within days, weeks, or months. These reasons are illogical and can lead physicians to act inhumanely, yet they are strong guiding considerations for many physicians. Betty and her two children, her son Chris and her daughter Candy (my wife), remembered Bud's experience all too vividly. They were shaken by it and were left with an abhorrence for the futile prolongation of life and for unnecessary suffering in the imminently dying.

After Bud's death in 1981, Candy had been a social worker on a hospice unit in a Minneapolis hospital. She was familiar with the compassion and appropriate care that can be given to dying patients by experienced and well-trained professionals. She often contrasted the senselessness of Bud's last days with her hospice experiences in Minneapolis.

Betty was an independent woman with strong feelings on many issues. She did not want to experience a prolonged, debilitating physical and mental deterioration as she died. She also did not want to become a burden to her family, and she had made extensive arrangements to ensure that a prolonged illness would not cause them any financial burden. She had worked hard to ensure that a reasonable estate would be left to her children upon her death.

Within a week of the diagnosis, Betty reacted to the situation in a way that surprised and hurt her children and is, to this day, difficult to explain. She withdrew, both physically and mentally, from her life and her family. She essentially went to her bedroom in her home and never came out again except for visits to the hospital and outpatient x-ray treatments.

An experienced ethics consultant, I now found myself deeply, emotionally involved in an ethical situation. I asked myself the same questions any ethics consultant would ask in a similar situation. Then I tried to examine how my answers and reactions might be affected because of my personal involvement. I evaluated Betty's case, using the same ethical framework that I had used on so many previous occasions. I decided that in many respects this would be an easy case to deal with.

First, I considered the medical condition and prognosis. Betty clearly had a terminal disease, with death likely within months and little chance for longer survival. She was not suffering a great deal physically at the time except for the unpleasant and uncomfortable swelling of her face. But this was a disease that could result in significant physical and mental suffering in the months ahead.

Second, I considered the benefits and burdens of medical treatment and alternative therapies. Nothing could result in a cure in Betty's case. The surgeon had done only a biopsy and did not attempt to remove the large malignant mass in her lung. The major therapeutic objectives were prolongation of some quality of life as judged by what the patient and her family wanted and the relief of pain and suffering.

For example, it was decided to give a course of radiation to the lung mass, not because it would cure but because it could result in some prolongation of life; more important, it could shrink the tumor, which would relieve pressure on the superior vena cava and decrease the swelling in her face. A combination of radiation and andiedema agents was effective in reducing the facial swelling.

Third, I considered Betty's wishes. In numerous conversations with her children and others over the years she had made clear how she would want to be treated in the event of a serious life-threatening illness. Perhaps she had made these wishes clear again when she went into her bedroom and withdrew from everyone. The family couldn't be sure. Perhaps they should have considered her withdrawal as a situational depression and sought professional advice. But her family felt that this withdrawal was probably a reflection of Betty's real thoughts and feelings: she was telling us what she wanted done. Because of this withdrawal, Betty did not engage in any significant conversations with her family about her current condition and treatment plan. Numerous attempts by her family and others to draw Betty out were unsuccessful.

Fourth, I evaluated the family's ability to render a responsible opinion regarding Betty's care. In my opinion, there was nothing ethically problematic here. This was a loving, caring family who had Betty's best interests at heart and wanted to act in accordance with her previously expressed wishes. A critical issue here and one that may become increasingly important in the future is family motivation. Physicians and other health care providers are often put in the uncomfortable position of evaluating the motivations of the family when prolonged treatment (whether beneficial or futile) or prolonged hospitalization or nursing care placement could have a devastating financial impact on the family, or when a substantial estate is involved. How far should health care professionals or ethics consultants go in evaluating the family's motivations? Should we attempt to discover the financial implications for family members of a patient's dying sooner or later? As technology becomes ever more sophisticated and ever more expensive, this issue may become more salient. Should the financial burden for the family ever be a morally relevant consideration in stopping treatment? This is a delicate and complex problem.

Fifth, I considered the opinions of the physicians and other health care providers involved in Betty's case. This is the area that Candy and I feared would present the greatest obstacle to Betty's humane care during her dying days. Unfortunately, we were correct.

In many ethical dilemmas the most critical factor blocking a satisfactory resolution of a case is communication—between physicians and family, between patients and family, among family members, or between the primary attending physician and other health care professionals. One of the most valuable functions of an ethics consultant is to facilitate communication among the primary decision makers: patient, family, and physician. For example, an ethics consultant may suggest a care conference if it is suspected that a major problem may be lack of communication. Bringing together the principal parties in a care conference, where everyone can speak freely and openly and share their concerns, feelings, doubts, and anxieties, can be one of the most satisfying aspects of an ethics consultation.

In this case, there was not a close trusting relationship between Betty and her physician. Because of her previous experience with the physician who cared for Bud in his final days and who did not keep his promise of adequately treating her father's suffering, Candy had serious reservations about how her mother would be treated, even though physicians are generally better at dealing with dying patients now than in the early 1980s. Candy was afraid she would let her mother down as she died, as she thought she had done with her father.

Only four weeks after the initial diagnosis, Betty was readmitted to the hospital because of confusion, hallucinations, and difficulty walking. A CAT scan of the brain revealed several tumor metastases. One of the physicians caring for Betty, an oncologist, informed Candy of this finding and then said, without discussing any alternatives, "We want to do radiation to the brain." My wife, the seasoned, experienced hospice worker, who knew very well her mother's strong feelings against futile treatment, said unhesitatingly, "You bet." After all, this was her mother, not a patient, and Candy reacted emotionally and instantly to the physician's only recommendation. This interchange and Candy's reaction demonstrates the powerful and intimidating influence of physicians on medical decision making.

Candy, who was at the hospital in Florida with her mother when informed of this diagnosis and the recommended treatment, called me immediately in Minneapolis. Candy and I had had several conversations about the likelihood of metastases throughout the body, especially to the brain; about how such a development would change our thinking, even about the short-term prognosis; and whether any treatment should be continued to maintain some acceptable quality of life in the presence of metastases. When Candy called me in Minneapolis, my response was, "Well now, wait a minute. Is this really what you and your mother want?" After reflecting on this for just a moment, Candy replied, "Of course, it's not what we want."

Within an hour of this conversation with Candy, I called the physician who had recommended radiation to the brain. Betty's prognosis was now significantly worse. On the basis of this new development, I told him that not only did we not want radiation to the brain, we also wanted to stop any further radiation treatments to the chest. When I told him what we had decided, which went against his recommendation of only a few hours ago, I expected some resistance, some comment or expression of displeasure or irritation that we were not following his suggested treatment. In fact, his only reply was "That's exactly what I would want done if it were me." If that's what he would have wanted done if it were he, then why didn't he suggest that to Candy? I didn't ask him.

At the beginning of this entire process I knew how strongly Candy and her mother felt about needless and unwanted suffering, especially at the hands of physicians who would not adequately address the suffering. Candy wanted to make sure that what had happened to Bud in 1981 didn't happen again with her mother. So I knew from the beginning that, when the end was near, we would take whatever steps were necessary and give whatever doses of pain medication were needed to treat Betty's suffering—physical and psychological. This goal was consistent with what I had taught for ten years in a biennial course in medical ethics with Jim Nelson, a dear friend and professional colleague, with the advice and recommendations of our ethics committee, to health care providers and families who sought our assistance on similar cases, and with what I had done over the years in my own personal practice.

The major practical problem for knowledgeable physicians is not the adequate treatment of suffering, it is knowing with some degree of reasonable certainty when the end is near—when Betty would become so critically ill that there would be no point in continuing any medication that would prolong her life. Principles are easy to articulate, but applying them in individual cases can be difficult. Betty's rapid downhill course and the brain metastases made it easier to determine when she was imminently dying. She would die within a few weeks, not a few months or longer as we had originally thought.

When Betty's diagnosis of cancer was initially made, I asked myself if there would be any circumstances in which I would consider active euthanasia as a last desperate resort, as the only means to relieve her suffering? The answer was no. As a physician and as an ethics consultant, I have never committed nor recommended active euthanasia. I have been in practice for eighteen years and have had only one serious request for active euthanasia—many years ago when a loving, caring son felt that his critically ill mother, who had suffered for years from parkinsonism and had sustained severe brain damage secondary to a respiratory arrest, had suffered enough.

Would I find it difficult to draw the lines between treating suffering and killing in Betty's case? Again, the answer was clearly no. There is almost always a well-demarcated line between the two, both in theory and in clinical practice. Betty would receive medications sufficient to keep her comfortable, even if those medications induced coma.

Candy and I were faced with the problem of who could manage Betty's case as she lay dying. We knew who could best make sure that Betty was treated well. We asked about a hospice nurse to care for Betty in her home, and we were extremely fortunate to find one. She was a typical hospice nurse: sensitive, caring, overworked, emotionally drained from caring for terminally ill patients and putting her head and heart into their care, full of common sense and wisdom, and frustrated by her frequent encounters with physicians who didn't seem to understand how to care humanely for the dying patient.

Stanva was magnificent. She was always available when we needed her. She gave us good advice about how to handle the physicians so as not to "irritate" them but yet get what we needed in terms of enough morphine on a prn (as needed) basis. Stanva really cared. Once we called her to complain that one of the practical nurses caring for Betty didn't seem to understand the medications she was giving to Betty. Stanva, who had a bad cold, had stayed home from work. Considering how sick she sounded, we asked if she could just make a phone call to Betty's house; that was all we expected. A few hours later, Stanva called us from Betty's house. As sick as she was, she had gone there, talked to the practical nurse, and straightened out the problem. That one episode illustrates her dedication.

As Betty's end drew near, Candy and I had great confidence that we had made the right choice of a capable health care professional to help her. The last two days of Betty's life, Stanva was always there when we needed her and when Betty need her. We talked frequently on the phone about Betty's care and about the exact doses and routes of medication to keep her comfortable. What do most patients and families do without a caring experienced hospice nurse like Stanva? The answer is not reassuring.

This was a unique case for me—to be so personally involved and yet to function as an ethics consultant. There was one area in which I felt very involved personally in which I think I was useful as an ethics consultant. Candy had a great fear that when the end was near, Betty would suffer needlessly and intensely, as her father had. I could see the look in Candy's eyes when she thought of that terrible possibility. Her feelings and fears affected me deeply; I didn't want to let Candy down, just as she didn't want to let Betty down when she was needed the most. My skills as an ethics consultant were most useful in making sure that Betty's dying process would be as comfortable and as dignified as possible. We feared that the main obstacle to this would be the attitudes and practices of the Winter Park physicians. The more we could remove the control of the dying process from the physicians, the more we could be assured that Betty's final days would be peaceful. I believe my skills as an ethics consultant were most helpful in encouraging the Winter Park physicians to give as much discretion as possible to Stanva, who could follow Betty's medical condition closely during her dying days and administer medications when appropriate.

There sometimes is a fine line between acting in a professional, composed manner and letting one's feelings express themselves in tragic situations. Patients, families, and health care professionals expect professionalism from ethics consultants, but they also appreciate knowing that consultants have feelings too. I can remember many times when, in talking with families, my eyes would start to get moist and my voice would begin to quiver and trail off. But I have never been ashamed of those times nor regretted that my emotions were manifesting themselves.

At the outset of this case, I wondered how often I would lose composure and what others would expect from me, being so intimately involved in a situation where I was also functioning as an ethicist. Surprisingly, I retained more composure than I thought I would. Sometimes, however, emotions can build up inside you. If these emotions are not released in some way, they may come out all at once. This is something I have learned over the years as an ethics consultant: to be aware of my emotions and allow them to be expressed, rather than have them build up and then be released in an inappropriate way or inappropriate time.

My immediate loyalty was to my wife, and I had to support her through this process, so I kept my emotions in check much of the time. One day, however, when Candy and I were talking on the phone (Candy in Florida and I in Minneapolis), all of the emotions that had been contained over the past few weeks released themselves, and for no apparent reason I started crying uncontrollably. Our conversation at that time was on a rather routine matter, so Candy was alarmed at my reaction, thinking that something else was wrong. She kept asking, "What's wrong, Ron, what's wrong?" I couldn't tell her because I was crying too hard. When something like that happens, I think it is best to get your emotions out, and that is exactly what I did—although I certainly scared my wife in the process.

On Tuesday night, June 16, Betty's condition worsened. She seemed more confused. She had been sleeping a great deal more, often throughout the day and night. The doctors had previously prescribed lorazepam for sedation, but the hospice worker and I now felt that morphine would be more appropriate. It would be just as effective in treating her suffering, but not nearly as sedating or as depressing to the respiratory system as lorazepam. Just as important, the doctors could prescribe larger standing orders for morphine than for lorazepam, allowing the hospice nurse and myself greater discretion in giving morphine when needed and increasing the amount as necessary. With standing orders from the physician, we would be able to use up to 240 mg of morphine every twenty-four hours.

Betty was taking many other medications for other medical problems. Because of my knowledge of these other medications and because of my status as a professional colleague of the physicians in Florida, I called her physician Wednesday morning and "suggested" changes in medications, doses, and route of administration, which the doctor promptly agreed to without hesitation. Throughout the entire process, I kept wondering what people do who don't have a physician (or an ethics consultant) in the family who can give this type of advice. The patient and family are usually at the mercy of physicians, who often have neither the time nor the motivation to care for their patients as I did for my mother-in-law. Would there be any doubt that most families would have readily acquiesced to the brain radiation after the recommendation of the doctor? How many families would have been able to stand up to a physician and say, "We appreciate your advice, but we don't think this treatment is going to give our mother any more meaningful life"?

Betty had been taking Decadron®, an antiedema drug used to treat swelling both of the face (from the venous obstruction in the chest) and of the brain (from the brain metastases). I now recommended that the Decadron be stopped. That would allow the brain swelling to increase, probably causing Betty to fall into a coma. Falling into a coma in a situation like this is usually painless, but we were running a slight risk that stopping the Decadron would allow the facial swelling to increase markedly without necessarily allowing coma to occur. An increase in facial swelling might cause a great deal of suffering for Betty and her family.

Did stopping the Decadron "hasten" Betty's death? Of course it did. Isn't hastening death the same as active euthanasia? Of course not. It is common practice for physicians to stop medications and allow patients to die, thereby "hastening" their deaths by minutes, hours, days, or even longer. But stopping treatment and allowing the underlying disease process to run its course and cause the death of the patient is radically different from administering a lethal dose of medication whose only purpose is to cause death directly.

In Betty's case, stopping the Decadron would probably hasten her death more than giving morphine. Stanva and I both knew that giving morphine in gradually increasing doses would result in significant relief of suffering without significant depression of respiration or consciousness. Thus, the administration of morphine in this case, even in massive doses, would not be active euthanasia. First, there would be a wide margin between the amount necessary for analgesia and the amount required for causing death through respiratory depression. Second, and just as important, our intent was only to give whatever dose was necessary to relieve suffering, not to kill.

All medications, except those for comfort, were stopped on Wednesday, June 18. Early Wednesday evening, Candy, Stanva, and I decided to give Betty an initial dose of 20 mg of morphine rectally. Candy and I were in Minneapolis, so the phone calls to Florida were frequent and long. Betty seemed very sedated after this initial dose, so, after further phone calls and discussion, we decided to give her only 10 mg rectally at 11 P.M. Our goal was not to cause coma or respiratory depression, only to keep her relatively sedated and without suffering. After stopping the Decadron, it could have taken a few days or longer before she would have gone into a coma from the swelling of her brain. So we expected that Betty would probably live a few more days, perhaps longer.

On Thursday, June 19, another 10 mg morphine was given rectally at 3 A.M. At this time, Betty did not appear to be suffering. At 6 A.M., we received a phone call from Winter Park; Betty had died at 5:30 A.M., less than twenty-four hours after most of her medications had been stopped and less than twelve hours after the morphine had been started.

Later we found out that Betty had complained to her practical nurse of mild chest pain on Wednesday afternoon. The autopsy revealed pneumonia as the immediate cause of death. The timing of the medication withdrawal and initiation of morphine had been much more fortuitous than we had realized at the time. Betty had not suffered from this pneumonia, a pneumonia that we would not have treated (unlike some terminally ill cancer patients who are treated time and time again in the final phases of their illness). Candy was relieved that her mother had not suffered. She had not let her mother down as she felt she had let her father down.

As Candy and I have looked back on this process, we have never had any doubts that we treated Betty the way Betty would have wanted to be treated. This was a quality-of-life decision, based on what the patient herself would have wanted. Betty would have been proud of her daughter and maybe of her son-in-law/physician/ethics consultant.

Some may question my involvement and influence in this case. Were the major decisions truly a reflection of Betty's wishes? Or were some decisions unduly influenced by my professional views (and personal biases and prejudices) as an ethics consultant? This concern could be raised in any case involving an ethics consultant and certainly in a situation in which the consultant is personally involved. In response to this legitimate concern, I can say two things. First, as in any ethics consultation that I do, I tried to be as aware as possible of the interplay between my professional–personal views (and my strengths and weaknesses as an ethics consultant) and the facts and circumstances of the case. Second, one would have to know the key players in this drama— Betty, Candy, other family members, Stanva, the doctors in Winter Park, and myself—and our interactions to judge whether my influences were appropriate.

Some might argue that what was done in this case was controversial and bordered on active euthanasia. That would be incorrect ethical judgment. We (those who cared for Betty in the last six weeks of her life) are proud of what we did. In my view, it is the way almost all terminally ill patients would want to be treated in their dying days, an ideal toward which others should strive. If all dying patients were treated similarly, there would be much less grass roots pressure toward legalizing active euthanasia.

Epilogue

WHAT do the cases in this book tell us about the process of ethics consultation, and what do they tell us about the practice of modern-day medicine?

Before addressing either of these questions, a few words about the cases the authors selected: Most of the ethical dilemmas described are typical. Experienced consultants have encountered variations of them many times. In ten of the twelve cases the central issue was whether and how a patient should be allowed to die. That ratio seems representative. However, eleven of the twelve patients had died by the end of the essay. That seems unrepresentatively high. Finally, in almost half of these cases the ethics consultation, though it was of some use, did not help bring about a clear resolution of the problem for which it was sought. Despite the consultant's intervention, the case dragged on and on until it was finally ended by the patient's death. That certainly happens occasionally, but more often a consultant can help catalyze a moral consensus about how to proceed that all parties find reasonable, and the case is satisfactorily resolved. These cases are atypical in their high degree of irresolution.

It is not surprising that many authors picked difficult and sometimes inconclusive cases about dying patients. These are the cases one remembers and thinks about for a long time. I would probably have picked such a case to write about myself. And there may be more to learn about medicine and about ethics consultation from these hard cases than from straightforward ones that a consultant manages expeditiously.

The Process of Ethics Consultation

Ethics consultation is a new field. There is as yet no agreed-on definition of its scope or constituent activities. One fact about ethics consultation, shown many times in the preceding pages, is that it involves more than consultation about ethics. Occasionally, ethical analysis does play the predominant role. Gert's case was like that: he explained to a patient's family why so many health care workers make an important distinction between active and passive euthanasia, and he clarified for them the underlying nature of that distinction. His analysis was sufficiently persuasive that the family no longer questioned the treatment plan being followed.

The consultants in this book, however, all did more than offer ethical opinions. Sometimes they evaluated the information given them, concluded that not enough of the morally relevant facts were known, and therefore encouraged further data collection. Brody, for example, believed his patient's neurological prognosis had not been sufficiently investigated and that important issues could not be resolved without that information. Some consultants, to obtain more data, talked directly to patients themselves, often to ascertain competent patients' preferences about the options open to them (Youngner, Bernat). Other consultants interviewed family members, usually to try to determine what an incompetent patient's values and preferences had been (Fletcher and Eulie).

Frequently the authors played a more active role than simply gathering data. Some held meetings with staff members to attempt to open up lines of communication or to resolve disagreements (Kopelman, Fleischman, Purtilo, Golenski, Nelson and Pomerantz). Others did even more: they became major participants as a case unfolded. Youngner, for example, became a kind of case manager, brokering information among disputing parties, even intervening with a recalcitrant resident. Two other authors entered into a case directly and assertively: Nelson, who encouraged a father to transfer his infant son to another hospital, and Cranford, who, along with a hospice nurse, managed the final days of his mother-in-law's life in her own home, partly out of exasperation with the attending physician (though neither of these two authors were acting as consultants to the patient's physician).

Two other features of the consultation process stand out in these essays. Once the necessary data are available, consultants usually do have opinions about what actions would and would not be morally appropriate in a particular case. That may surprise some persons. There is a mistaken view about applied ethics that the field cannot arrive at any answers, that the best it can do is to clarify the reasons for and against acting in various ways, and that choosing any option then becomes a purely subjective matter.

But applied ethics is much more objective than that. Once the facts about a case are known and agreed on, there is, more often than not, a general consensus about what actions would and would not be morally appropriate. It is a truism among ethics consultants that a dilemma initially presented as a disagreement about values usually turns out to be a disagreement about facts. Some general issues are intractable— abortion is the best example—but most specific cases that are referred to ethics consultants are not. That is why the consultants in this book rarely appeared to be tongue-tied, or to be only contemplative and discursive in their approach.[1]

But if applied ethics is reasonably precise and rigorous, the field of medical ethics consultation is still feeling its way. In part this is because the field does involve more than conceptualization. It is not enough to be adept in applying theory to facts; it is also necessary to know how to obtain additional facts, how to talk with interested parties who may disagree among themselves, and how to conduct oneself as a new participant entering a case, a new participant who usually has some credibility but rarely has any power. The field is evolving; that is apparent in the self-critical remarks made by many authors in this book. Some of the most experienced ethics consultants in the country have written here, but several of them thought by the end of their case that they should have done some things significantly differently.

Ethics consultants fill a new role in American medicine, a fascinating role that blends the ethical, the psychological, and the interpersonal. That there is such a role to fill, particularly in the setting of the dying patient, says a great deal about modern medical practice.

Dying in America

When I initially read these essays, I wondered what impression they would give a lay reader about medical practice in America. I wondered in particular what impression they would give of dying in American hospitals, since so many of the authors wrote about that topic. I think they give a rather bad impression but not a wholly inaccurate one.

There are examples in these stories of doctors who act sensitively and judiciously toward gravely ill patients and their families. But there are also examples of physicians who are a part—sometimes the major part—

of the problem the ethics consultant confronts. Some physicians in this book seem unable to talk in a straightforward manner to dying patients or their families. Others overtreat dying patients, and some of these, one eventually finds out, have been distorting the facts and presenting a falsely optimistic prognosis to the family. Most generally, many of these physicians seem unable to formulate a rational care plan to guide their decisions over time; rather, their cases seem to putter along from day to day until some crisis forces the next move.

It would be incorrect to think that most physicians are as uncommunicative or as faltering as some of the physicians in these essays. In fact I worry that this book gives too negative an impression of doctors. I worry specifically that the doctors who read this book may keep at arm's length from ethics consultants for fear of being exposed as inept! That would be an unfortunate result. Most of the doctors in my hospital manage dying patients competently, and in my experience doctors who request ethics consultations are usually among the most ethically sensitive of all physicians. Having made these qualifications, it would be naive not to acknowledge that all too many physicians do not handle this part of their practice well. Some of them handle it quite poorly.

Why do some physicians do such a bad job? One problem is that some doctors have an overweening bias toward keeping patients alive as long as possible. There is less of this than there was a decade ago, but it is still present. Of course for doctors to "err" in the direction of preserving life is not a bad thing; most of us would want our doctors, if unsure, not to allow death to come too soon. But the bias I'm describing goes beyond that; it is an inclination to use any life support and to press for any treatment that keeps a body alive. This is the "Death is the enemy; anytime a patient of mine dies I take it as a personal failure!" approach.

There is a less extreme version of this attitude, which is seen more frequently. Some doctors, though they disapprove in theory of overtreating the dying, are reluctant to withdraw life support unless they feel certain there is no legal jeopardy in doing so. In some hospitals this attitude is encouraged by the hospital's lawyer(s), who may feel that they should minimize any and all exposure to legal liability. I have heard people say, "Nobody ever got sued for keeping a patient alive." In fact, this is no longer true: suits are beginning to be filed for unwanted overtreatment. Even the underlying fear is nearly groundless; suits against a physician for allowing a gravely ill patient to die sooner rather than later are almost nonexistent.

If any legal uncertainty exists, however, a doctor's and a hospital's response is often simply to allow treatment to continue. This sometimes represents not so much a positive decision to continue to treat as an unwillingness to make any decision other than to keep doing what is already being done. There is a difference between these two positions: one can openly debate a clear decision either to continue treating or not to continue treating, but it is harder to debate the nondecision of simply letting the status quo persist. Frequently, there is no trenchant discussion of any kind; rather, the case simply drags on. The patient, if not totally unconscious, continues to suffer to a greater or lesser degree. Finally, as in the cases in this book, the patient almost always dies. The patient has gained nothing and may have lost a lot; but the doctor and the hospital have not had to worry overmuch about a lawsuit, and no one needs to feel afterward that less than everything possible was done. None of this is to suggest anything other than aggressive treatment when a nontrivial chance of recovery exists *and* when one believes a formerly competent patient would have wanted treatment under the present circumstances. But in so many of these treat-and-treat cases these conditions do not exist.

In most of the cases in this book there was not only uncertainty about whether a patient should be allowed to die sooner rather than later, there was disagreement. Sometimes (as in the Fletcher and Eulie and Golenski cases) the family wanted more treatment than the health care team thought warranted, sometimes (as in Nelson and in Youngner) the family wanted less, and sometimes (as in Kopelman) the staff itself was significantly divided.

That doctors frequently press for more treatment than either a family or a patient desires will not be news to most of the readers of this book. What is less widely appreciated is how often families insist, even in hopeless situations, that "everything possible" be done. Their motives are kind, but the results often are not. They say: "I could never live with myself if we didn't try everything"; "Miracles do happen—I read about one just last week"; "I'll get a lawyer and sue this hospital for everything it's worth if you even think of letting my mother die." This last remark, especially, almost always chills both physician and hospital, and treatment goes on. If the patient is unconscious, perhaps little is wasted except money and resources. But if the patient, though incompetent, is still conscious, much unnecessary suffering may occur.

Because of our ever-increasing technological sophistication, dilemmas and disagreements about allowing patients to die are frequent.

They will surely become more frequent in the future. Bodies can be kept alive for a long time. Even in situations where further treatment or life support seems pointless to most observers, including most family members, it is always possible for one person, out of sincerely benevolent motives, to wish to continue. And there are many cases in which further treatment would not be totally pointless but in which the patient, were he or she competent to decide, would not want further treatment at all. Talk to a group of senior citizens and ask them how many would want a long course of aggressive treatment if the chance of significant recovery were 10 percent or less, with a great likelihood that even if they did recover they would have significant residual handicaps as a result of their illness. A very few say they want to be treated given that scenario, but the great majority, in my experience, do not.

Managing One's Own Dying

Some readers may be distressed by the cases described in this book and wonder what they can do to avoid these situations. How can lay persons increase the control they have over how and when they will be allowed to die? How can overtreatment at the end of life be avoided, whether the impetus to overtreatment comes from one's doctor or one's family? It seems appropriate to end this epilogue and this book with some discussion of these issues. There are at least two steps that can be taken.

First, all adults should record their wishes about dying in some form of "advance directive." A Living Will can be signed and a Durable Power of Attorney for Health Care can be drawn up, whether or not one lives in a state where these documents have been given explicit legal sanction by the state legislature. Living Wills typically have a prewritten text stating that if the signer of the document becomes terminally ill and permanently incompetent he or she would not want life support to be continued. Durable Powers of Attorney for Health Care are more robust and flexible. They allow the signers to appoint agents to make health care decisions for them should they become incompetent to make them for themselves.

One can write into the text of a Durable Power of Attorney specific instructions about any of a number of contingencies: whether to continue life support in the event one is not terminally ill but is permanently unconscious;[2] whether, in addition to discontinuing other forms of life support in particular situations, one would also want artificial feeding to be discontinued; and whether, if one were gravely ill, one would always want to be treated until the situation became completely hopeless.[3] Being specific about these matters not only gives useful direction to one's family and one's health care team, it assuages much of the worry about litigation that infects doctors and hospitals.[4,5]

A second important step is to discuss, ahead of time, these documents and the instructions they contain with pertinent family members and with one's primary care physician. That not only decreases the chance of future misunderstandings or ambiguities, it allows one to determine whether any of these individuals might object to following one's instructions. The person one appoints as an agent in a Durable Power of Attorney for Health Care, for example, should feel comfortable with the instructions he or she may be asked to carry out in the future. But one's physician should be queried as well. If a person directed, for example, that if she became permanently unconscious she would want all life support to be withheld or withdrawn, including, if necessary, all food and fluids, then she should make certain that her primary care physician would be willing to follow these instructions should that situation arise. If her physician for any reason would not, then she must decide what to do. One option, if these matters are sufficiently important to her, is to find another primary care physician who would be willing to follow her instructions.

Modern life-support technology has forced on our generation the necessity of making more fine-grained decisions about the management of our dying than has ever previously been the case. It is not *necessary* to make these decisions; death will eventually come whether we make them or not. But we may spare ourselves and our loved ones considerable physical pain and mental anguish if we reflect on these matters and record our wishes while we are still able to do so.

Notes

1. I am offering conclusions here about the objectivity of ethics, but I am not giving supporting arguments. Interested readers may wish to consult Bernard Gert, *Morality* (New York: Oxford University Press, 1988), 48–49, 258–60.

2. Karen Ann Quinlan and Nancy Cruzan are widely publicized examples of patients in this category.

3. Charles M. Culver, "On Managing One's Own Dying," *Social Responsibility: Business, Journalism, Law, Medicine* 15 (1989): 5–15.

4. For information about advance directives specific to one's own state of residence, write to National Council on Death and Dying, 250 West 57th Street, New York, NY 10107. (This is a new organization recently formed by the merger of

Concern for Dying and the Society for the Right to Die.) For a general discussion of advance directives, including a list of suggested questions to answer in a Durable Power of Attorney for Health Care, see Culver, "On Managing One's Own Dying," and Charles M. Culver and Bernard Gert, "Beyond the Living Will: Making Advance Directives More Useful," *Omega* (1990, in press).

5. The June 25, 1990, U.S. Supreme Court decision in the Nancy Cruzan case makes clear that the U.S. Constitution permits a person to refuse life-support, and the Court made no distinction between refusing artificial feeding and refusing other forms of life-sustaining treatment. The Court did allow individual states, however, if they wished, to demand clear and convincing evidence that a currently unconscious patient would in fact have wanted particular forms of life-support to be withdrawn. This ruling underscores the importance of filling out advance directives, and filling them out with the requisite degree of specificity.